MW01278454

Naturally There's Hope

A Handbook for the Naturopathic Care of Cancer Patients

Dr. Neil McKinney, B.Sc., R.Ac., N.D.

© Copyright 2003 Neil McKinney. All rights reserved.

No part of this publication may be reproduced, stored in a retrieval system, or transmitted, in any form or by any means, electronic, mechanical, photocopying, recording, or otherwise, without the written prior permission of the author.

Printed in Victoria, Canada

National Library of Canada Cataloguing in Publication Data

McKinney, Neil, 1952-
    Naturally, there's hope : a handbook of naturopathic cancer care / Neil McKinney.

Includes bibliographical references and index.
ISBN 1-4120-0464-0

    1. Cancer--Alternative treatment. 2. Naturopathy. I. Title.

RZ440.M355 2003   616.99'406   C2003-903814-9

TRAFFORD

This book was published on-demand in cooperation with Trafford Publishing.
On-demand publishing is a unique process and service of making a book available for retail sale to the public taking advantage of on-demand manufacturing and Internet marketing. On-demand publishing includes promotions, retail sales, manufacturing, order fulfilment, accounting and collecting royalties on behalf of the author.

Suite 6E, 2333 Government St., Victoria, B.C. V8T 4P4, CANADA
Phone   250-383-6864   Toll-free 1-888-232-4444 (Canada & US)
Fax   250-383-6804   E-mail   sales@trafford.com
Web site   www.trafford.com TRAFFORD PUBLISHING IS A DIVISION OF TRAFFORD HOLDINGS LTD.
Trafford Catalogue #03-0833   www.trafford.com/robots/03-0833.html

10   9   8   7   6   5

Dedication

To my darling wife Lynda I dedicate this project.

You want to live in good health to 100 years old. I want to spend all of that and more with you.

With your support I eat well, and have balance and love in my life.

You are my right arm as office manager of our Vital Victoria Naturopathic Clinic.

You are a Reiki healer and wise crone.

I have studied and collected all the best ideas I can find to prevent cancer and to treat cancer patients. Thanks to your support this work can now offer hope for improved life and living
to all of us.

Bless you.

Naturally There's Hope
A Handbook for the Naturopathic Care of Cancer Patients

Dr. Neil McKinney, BSc,RAc,ND

Table of Contents

Chapter Twenty-Two - <u>Research Mehods & Scientific Evidence</u>

Introduction -   A JOURNEY TO HEALING

I was born with the help of a nurse midwife at Vancouver General Hospital.
The doctor never did show up. Alternative medicine is the story of my life.

I had an epiphany at age 15 which made me aware that there was more to healing,
beyond drug medicine. I had the misfortune to suffer a very severe burn to my right foot,
stepping into a bed of coals in a beach fire pit. The injury was extreme, and was
complicated by a delay of 4 days to get from the isolated West coast of Vancouver Island
to a hospital, in the town of Hope, B.C.   I was given Codeine for pain, which I took
only once – the effect it had on my psyche was worse than the physical pain.

On returning home, I was offered help from a man I knew well, who was like a surrogate
father to me. I loved and respected this fellow as a wholesome role model of a loving
family man. I was very surprised to be told he did "faith healing". I was not sure I had
the same faith he had, but he said it was not religious, and in any case he had enough
faith for both of us. I was being told by the physicians I could lose my foot, so it was a
no-brainer to say yes.   He did a simple technique of non-touch healing, holding his
hands beside my upper neck until he felt the skull and upper neck bones line up, then
held a hand over the top of my head and the other over my poor foot. I could feel
something odd moving around, and a distinct warmth. I was nearly all healed in 3 days!
I have no scars or signs to show the foot was ever injured. This was truly miraculous!
My physician could not grasp what he was seeing when I showed him the suddenly
improved foot. He actually scolded me and threw me out of his office, convinced I was
my twin brother playing a prank on him - but he knew we are fraternal twins and don't
actually look alike! The poor fellow had the same reaction most men of science and
learning have to evidence of energetic healing - he denied the facts before his very eyes. I
could not, and so learned the technique, which I have used on a few occasions with
powerful results. He attributed this method to a Japanese teacher or *sensei*.   I see it as
being related to the popular technique of Reiki healing.

I was fascinated by reports about acupuncture and Traditional Chinese Medicine (TCM)
that surfaced in the media in 1972 after the American President Richard Nixon went to
China. With normalization of relations between East and West came a significant
cultural exchange. China had one very unique and valuable export: its system of
Traditional Chinese Medicine (TCM). Seeing people getting major surgery while talking
to the surgeon, then getting up and walking back to their hospital room was completely
mind-boggling.

I thought to myself the Chinese are very smart, a whole lot of them have been using this type of medicine from time immemorial, so there just must be something to learn from them. I transferred out of the mathematics and physics program at Simon Fraser University (SFU), which was to take me into architecture and engineering. My new goal became to study Western medicine and then go on into TCM and acupuncture. I had the ambition to try to take the best of science and modern medicine and meld it with traditional and subtle forms of healing. I hoped to one day understand some of my unusual healing experiences from a rational point of view. I wanted the doctors and skeptics to grasp the potential in all of us to be healed. After finishing a pre-med bachelor degree in biology and biophysics, I worked awhile for the Dean of Sciences in biophysical research at SFU Biosciences.

I went on to apply to regular medical school, but found intolerant attitudes at the University of British Columbia (UBC) towards TCM and other alternative healing methods such as homeopathy. It was bluntly scornful and unwelcoming. I came to the conclusion that I was not one who could adapt to those arch-conservative attitudes. I imagined myself getting through all those years of study only to have the mind-control of the medical establishment turn on me and strip me of my hard-earned right to practice, or worse, turn me into yet another medical bigot. They had some things I wanted to study, but they did not have the wisdom to use the resources of the wider world of wholistic and traditional medicine and healing.

I decided to put some distance between me and my family and the school, and to rethink my direction. I did not understand the psychological process then in these terms, but I needed to set out on a traditional "vision quest" - to find a new direction for my life journey, assess the gifts given by Nature for my benefit and for that of others in my life, to determine what I was supposed to do with this life I have been blessed with, and to identify what resources and allies could help me achieve those goals.

I took a globe of the world and put one finger on Vancouver and the other on the opposite side of the planet. I was hoping it wasn't too cold there (please don't let it be Antarctica!). The spot turned out to be in the middle of the Indian Ocean. The nearest land was the Southern tip of India, so that is where I decided to go to ponder my next move. I took a train across Canada, flew from Montreal to London, England, and then to continental Europe to establish a base in Denmark. I took the infamous "Magic Bus" from Amsterdam to New Delhi, 40 days and nights to India. I left the European bus and took local transport from Kabul, Afghanistan by train, through Pakistan, to the Punjab. Next was New Delhi, Northern India, the Taj Mahal, South to Madras, eventually reaching the tip of the Indian subcontinent. I recall meditating at the Swami Yogananda Memorial Rock at Kanyakumari, relieved to be at this peaceful spot to reconstruct my life goals. Like so many Westerners, while in South India I fell very ill

with amoebic dysentery. Fortunately, I experienced an impressive rapid cure with homeopathic medicine. I was even more impressed when this remedy helped some fellow travellers who had the same condition and were not doing really well despite prescribed drug medicines. I went back to the Homeopathic Medical Doctor and with a translator asked what these amazing little sugar pills were. I was told they were a very dilute form of a medicine which could cause the same illness if taken in a big amount, but in the small dose helped the body to heal - something like a vaccination. I was OK to that point, but became upset and confused when told that the more it was diluted the stronger it became! I asked for the titles of any books that could help me understand this apparent paradox. The "boy-scientist" had his second transformational medical experience
- *a miraculous cure by an impossible medicine.*

On returning to Canada I worked a year as a laboratory instructor at the University of Victoria. I was in the microbiology department, working with 1st to 4th year science students and nurses. I ran the lab, grew the bacteria, made sure the experiments worked, and taught techniques such as disinfection and sterilization, culture of fastidious organisms, and so on. I liked the work, but the pay was terrible.

The next year I was working in the Medical Biophysics Unit of the B.C. Cancer Research Foundation as a research technician doing tissue culture. I grew human and animal cells in dishes in a lab, put them into an artificial gelatin tissue model I made, and did rather cruel things to them with radiation. I did refuse to do any experiments with mice or other animals. We were looking at a radiation sensitizing drug to enhance cancer radiotherapy, and a new form of radiation called *pi mesons* generated at the UBC nuclear particle cyclotron TRIUMF
(Tri-University Meson Factory).

While living in Langley, my daughter Angela was born, in our home with a midwife attending. I looked for a homeopathic doctor for my family, and found Dr. Robert Fleming, N.D., a naturopathic physician. To my delight, he was also a skilled acupuncturist and a homeopath. He suggested I become a naturopathic doctor, but I was enjoying my cancer research work, which I continued for over 5 years.

Who should walk into our cancer research laboratory one day, but Terry Fox!? I had seen him once before, running around the track at Simon Fraser University on his prosthetic leg. That hop-a-long gait of his was labored, but he did not accept it as a handicap. You had to admire his grit, and I recall saying hello as he passed.

I did not know then that he had lost his leg to cancer. He had been spending time with kids with cancer in local hospitals, giving them encouragement and support.
He decided he needed to do more to try to stop the hurting. He was planning to run across Canada to raise money for cancer research.

He stood in my laboratory and spoke softly and passionately about all the wonderful things "smart guys like you" would find to cure cancer, when enough Canadians got interested and gave enough money to the scientists. I thought he was a little naïve, but you had to try to believe along with him. We spoke a second time before his run began. That time we talked about investing more research dollars in new sources of ideas, by putting more funds into graduate students with fresh and original concepts and techniques.

I didn't want to knock the major research institutions, but there is a certain conservatism in the old-boy's network of peer review. Most of the money seemed to go to the "same old-same old". Scientists who did great and hard work as doctoral students often spun out their thesis work into a career of repeating much the same stuff until retirement. The well-ordered ranks of scientific medicine and medical research plod on, certain of the correctness of their theories and intent on doing the best thing. However, it is seldom the really large cancer institutions which innovate most of the major advances in this field. More often progress comes from the clinician or the novice scientist alert to the possibility of something really new. You see what you look for.

Terry was very focused on helping reduce the carnage from cancer. I was just in awe of his courage, optimism and humanity. Terry was forced to quit his run in Thunder Bay, Ontario. He came back to B.C. and announced his cancer had relapsed and he was medically unfit to continue his Marathon of Hope. When Terry passed away a few months later, I left research and entered naturopathic medical school. I decided I too could no longer wait passively for academia and pure science to muddle through to a cure for cancer. I needed to get in the trenches and help someone right away.
First, I toured some of the "alternative" cancer clinics in Southern California and across the border in Tijuana, Mexico. I took another year of university in health sciences, spent 4 years studying naturopathic medicine, and 3 years of acupuncture and TCM. I have practiced for about 18 years now. In the early years of practice I concentrated on helping support patients through radiation, surgery and chemotherapy. In this adjunctive role I did often succeed in getting things back onto the rails when the harsh medical treatment threatened to finish them before it had a chance to cure their cancer, or at least put it into remission. Real alternatives or a cure remained elusive.

It is only in the last few years that I feel I have finally begun to reach that goal set so long ago, to really help people with cancer with natural medicines. I have created some of my own protocols and formulas, and have found other doctors and scientists who have reached similar conclusions. Many of the therapies I use are becoming common among my peers in naturopathic medicine and of course many are very time-tested classical formulae from Traditional Chinese Medicine.

Few of these alternative approaches to cancer have had the benefit of controlled human trials. Scientific investigation and clinical research in cancer has largely focused on cytotoxic, patent protected synthetic drugs, radiation and surgery. Implicit in the natural approach is use of the extraordinary synergy of complex mixtures of herbs, antioxidants, and other natural bio-compatible agents. They are often seen as "crude drugs" in need of purification and concentration. Indeed, no single natural agent is of much use all on its own. The complexity of these biological medicines is a barrier to their scientific investigation under the old chemical drug model. Just because there has been no rush to fund the research to validate most natural therapies does not refute their value. It is always a subjective decision to apply a treatment, which may or may not be backed up by scientific data. There are no certainties in the practice of medicine. Each case is a dynamic and non-linear system with no certain outcome. The standard for selecting a therapy is an informed choice of utilitarian remedies which have a known favorable risk versus benefit ratio. Few synthetic drugs have truly high level proof of safety and efficacy. The research is just too expensive for the public system. Without drug company money, most natural products are not likely to ever be scientifically supported to the point that will satisfy the professional skeptics in academia. The prejudice against natural products in health care is economic and political. Whether there is a scientific basis for not using them is simply not known. Scientific conclusions are not drawn from experiments which have not been done.

Many natural therapies reported by clinicians to be active against cancers have been rejected after failing the National Cancer Institute's screening process for activity against a number of isolated cancer cell types in the laboratory. This strategy fits with the needs of drug companies for small synthesizable molecules which can become patentable drugs.

This strategy also assumes that the best approach to cancer cells is to directly kill them with cytotoxins (cell poisons). These molecules must be purified, analyzed, identified, and synthesized. The very suggestion of using whole plant extracts with multiple ingredients creates an immediate and insumountable impasse for the biochemists.

They cannot "characterize" the structure of every component and describe a molecular mechanism for the properties observed. Doctors are justifiably cautious about putting strange new synthetic molecules into the human body, but are they not disqualifying themselves from evaluating traditional medicines as they are traditionally used? Is it appropriate to even do experiments which disrupt the very process they are purporting to measure?

There are humane physicians around the world who integrate therapies such as diet, detoxification, exercise, emotional support, music, and spiritual practices. These greatly impact quality of life. They are very difficult to quantify, "unproven", but of course much sought after by patients. This is because *life has value*.

Natural therapies with plant medicines, living foods and nutritional supplements are rationally directed to immune strengthening, normalizing cell signalling, and encouraging bad cells to commit suicide (apoptosis). Scant resources have moved into place to screen for these properties in foods and plants. The National Institute of Health Office of Alternative Medicine research center has a budget of 0.005% of that of the National Cancer Institute. These remedies are much more complex than the medications in synthetic drug trials. Pure drugs have resulted in a lot of toxicity and little progress in curing cancer. It is time to reconsider the use of complex biological approaches from living sources, which evolution has experimented with and perfected over millions of years.

I participated in the Credentialling Committee of the Tzu Chi Institute of Complementary and Alternative Medicine (CAM) Research at Vancouver General Hospital. It is unfortunate that it is even more of an issue of *who* does the work rather than the merit of the work that is made the focus. The medical doctors don't want anyone else on their turf, and so they are generally unable to accept the value of natural medicine research done by anyone outside their fraternity. Again I ran into the brick wall of the UBC scientific review panels deciding CAM was not even worth researching. The Institute was never permitted to conduct a substantive program with a multidisciplinary input from the health professions licensed to practice complementary & alternative medicine. The Institute languished for years under the supervision of people who actually state it is "unethical" to do human research with unproven remedies - because they are unproven! Medicines which have been used by billions of folk, prescribed by millions of physicians, over thousands of years. Unproven? The Institute has now closed.

"If we knew what we are doing it wouldn't be called research"
Albert Einstein

It is considered ethical in cancer wards to continually research synthetic drugs never put in a human body in the prior course of history. Trials are going on all the time, and new combinations and doses are being tried all the time. Oncologists' expert opinions often do vary.

In fact only a small part of orthodox medical practice meets the standard of proven safety and effectiveness in large multi-centered double blind controlled studies.

Whether these ideas on the natural healing of cancer I present here are pre-scientific, rational, evidence-based, or beyond science depends on your point of view. Expert opinion does vary. The best and brightest, the most honorable and reputable of my peers use these medicines.

I am a steward of a body of knowledge which has good clinical outcomes in many areas of oncology. We get stabilization, responses, remissions, and qualitative improvements in many difficult cases. Why the science industry has ignored or overlooked some of these therapies I have been able to find, I cannot say. I have tried to sift the science from the nonsense, and to avoid the temptation to spin straw into gold. The result is a robust and comprehensive naturopathic oncology.

My experience says that patient-centered care needs to be multidimensional and multidisciplinary. Patients know this and are demanding it. They are paying for it privately, and getting it.

The naturopathic oncologist must integrate complementary and alternative medicine with that of other care-givers. It is clearly interdependent with orthodox medical and radiation oncology. Biological physicians add particular expertise in nutrition and dietetics, botanicals, psychology, and energetic healing. All naturopathic physicians licensed today have the medicine and skill to be able to profoundly improve the quality of life of any person with cancer. The *Vis medicatrix naturae* – the healing power of Nature - can relieve pain, detoxify, tonify and restore health.

Patients with cancer today need comfort, palliation, treatment and cures. They have been patiently waiting and hoping, and dying, while the wheels of the science industry turn without moving forward appreciably. There is safety in bio-compatible medicines derived from natural and living sources proven by traditional use. We know very well what they do to humans, and we are learning what they do to cancerous cells. Evidence from academic scientific research in test tubes, on animals, from observation and human experimentation, and from clinical practice, is moving natural medicine to the front-line in primary cancer care.

The war on cancer will begin to be won when nutritional and truly biological medicine is merged with the more common orthodox physical and chemical medicines. They are genuinely complementary. The modern diet has insufficient nutritional value in several key areas, creating and maintaining a cancer epidemic. We naturopathic doctors have a saying *We dig our graves with our knives and our forks.*

What we hope for is the day when we all know how to build our health and strength with living and natural foods.

We are told sun exposure on the skin is a major source of preventable cancer. We also know that vitamin D, when activated in the skin by ultraviolet light, helps calcium be absorbed from the gut and is also significantly protective against a wide variety of cancers. Now we are seeing a lot of Canadians showing up with rickets, osteomalacia (bone pain) and calcium disorders from lack of activated vitamin D due to avoidance of the sun. They are good citizens trying to avoid the sun and use high SPF sunscreen as advised by public health experts. What is wrong with our relationship to the sun? Is it the thinning ozone layer that is making the sun so dangerous? No, the answer is not out in the ozone. It is the lack of the light protectants from the aerial parts of plants which are deficient in our present diet. Most plants seek out direct sunlight, and have evolved defenses against ultraviolet ray damage. They can share these life-giving substances with us, just as they provide us with the only source of oxygen.

It seems they are perfect for us. Chlorophyll, flavenoids, polyphenols, isoflavones and antioxidants found in whole plant foods are the missing elements in our fight against skin and every other sort of cancer.

To our good fortune, these nutrients are also associated in wholesome foods with health and immune building compounds such as high fibre, omega 3 fatty acids, long chain polysaccharides, high potassium, high calcium, trace minerals, vitamin A, and a host of other natural healers. The food which got our ancestors through the millenia can also ensure our future.

Our ancestors rarely got cancer. Was the world perfect for them, or were they perfect for the world? Imagine having the robust strength of a caveman with the medicine to take care of his nemesis - infectious disease and traumatic injury. We have the genetics to be much healthier than we are. We need to develop a culture that sees past disease control to the higher state of real health. We also need "green" physicians who will stand up against the pollution of our bodies by man-made chemicals and environmental toxins. When governments move to restrict petrochemicals, cancer deaths are prevented. The best example of this was the banning of a handful of pesticides in Israel, with a subsequent drop in cancer rates of nearly 30% in a few years.

The general population no longer trusts scientists, government and organized medicine to put their safety ahead of financial and industrial interests. We are not content to be polluted and malnourished for profit, and forced to rely on the obviously inadequate medical system to correct the resulting disease.

I offer this summary of the state of naturopathic care of cancer to the suffering and mortal humanity that needs clinical help today. I hope that with professional guidance in applying them, the insights I present in this volume will have an impact on the health care of my community immediately.

We "nature doctors" have at the ready:
- alternatives for those who will not or cannot continue to take orthodox medical care.
- complementary care to support the allopathic approach, and make it more likely to succeed.
- an important role to play in prevention.

There is a great craving by the public for all the doctors and practitioners to work together. I have run a multidisciplinary clinic, and had a local medical doctor who wanted to work with me give up because his peers harassed him about it. I worked to get a multidisciplinary approach in the Tzu Chi institute for Complementary and Alternative Medicine Research, and saw the medical establishment kill that idea as well. I will not give up the vision of a unified system of *health* care. I now teach at a naturopathic medical school where all the professions work together, as they did where I trained in the United States. There are a few in each profession with vision, and who value diversity of opinions. We will see a day when rigorous scientific medicine in the Western model is just one of the tools for cancer. There is a time to slash and burn this horrid disease. However, it is also obvious to most people today that there is a place for gentler methods too, treating the mind, body and spirit.

We are free to choose our own path through this life. I believe we are gifted with the support we need to be healed. These are the plants and the foods - and each other - which Nature has put here with us. With all the forces of Nature at our disposal, naturally there's hope for better outcomes with cancer.

Chapter One -   CANCER BASICS

- In the USA in the year 2001 - over 1,300,000 new people were diagnosed with cancer; treatment costs were over $100 billion US dollars. Divide by 10 to get the Canadian figures.

- Cancers are the second leading cause of death.

- Cancer will affect 1 in 3 persons alive today, and about 1 in 5 will die of cancer.

- Cancers have 50% mortality, meaning half of those diagnosed with cancer will end up dying of that cancer, despite the very best of modern medical care.

- Cancer has very high morbidity, meaning it causes great sickness and harm, again despite the best of modern medical care. Is it any wonder sensible people are looking at alternatives in cancer care?

- People greatly fear both the disease and treatments. In fact nearly 100% of those diagnosed with cancer will suffer some harm from the treatment. They may be disfigured or maimed by the surgery, suffer various complications, be burned by the radiation and scar up, or be made very ill by the chemotherapy drugs. Orthodox treatment can kill patients, and it can trigger cancer cell formation, resulting years later in another cancer even if the first type was cured by the treatment. Is it any wonder sensible, educated and cautious people are using all possible adjuncts to reduce the harm from cancer therapy, to restore their full health, and to prevent a reoccurence?

- There are at least 300 distinct neoplastic diseases we call cancer. Cancer is not a simple disease, it has many forms, many causes, and therefore there is no simple cure. What works for one cancer at one stage in one person will not always do the same for another person, another cancer type, or the same cancer in the same person at a later stage.

- 10 % of deaths of children under age 15 are due to cancers, notably acute leukemias and brain tumors. Aging increases cancer risk.

- Most benign tumors do not become cancerous. However, if they get large in the wrong place they can be as damaging as cancer.

- Diagnosis is only certain from microscopic examination by a skilled scientist of tissues obtained by biopsy or surgical excision, needle aspiration, washings, cytological (cell) scrapings and smears. We do not treat cancer until it is confirmed by a trained and licensed pathologist looking at the stained cells magnified under a microscope!

- Epidemiology is the study of disease trends in large populations. It gives a way to sort out the multiple factors which act to create or prevent diseases. As an example, you can look at the occurrence of heart disease in those who smoke cigarettes and compare it to the rate for non-smokers, and you can see it is much worse in smokers. You can then tell a smoker how much risk they are taking by smoking. Since real individuals often do some things which are good and several things which are bad - at least bad for their biology – it is only by this method that the relative role of each action can be discerned. Epidemiology research into cancer has led many experts and textbooks to state that 'Remarkable differences can be found in the incidence and death rates of specific forms of cancer around the world'. The biggest differences arise from cultural factors, especially diet. Use of too many chemicals, occupational and environmental factors are clearly triggering certain cancers in certain populations.

The role of genetics in cancer is surprisingly minor, considering the central role of DNA abnormalities in cancer. Studies with twins show inherited factors increase risk for stomach, colorectal, lung, breast and prostate cancers by 26 to 42%. Certain races have increased risk of certain cancers, although it is really a saw-off as they often have lower risk from other conditions.

However, a whopping 70 to 90% of cases are attributable to environmental and cultural factors rather than genetic predisposition, and are therefore theoretically preventable. For example risk arises from exposure to *xenobiotics* - chemicals which accidently mimic our hormones, from man-made (exogenous) hormones, tobacco, alcohol, amines, polyamines, polycyclic aromatic hydrocarbons formed by burning sugars, excess sun exposure, heavy metals, pesticides, and excess sugar intake.

Asian women have low risk of breast cancer, but when they move to the USA and adopt the American diet and lifestyle their risk increases by 60%. Overall, immigrants to our Western civilization lifestyle see increased cancer risk of 80% after 10 years exposure.

What is really awful is that in our culture the risk of cancer is rising every year. All the well paid scientists regulating our food and water and air supply and purporting to keep us safe are obviously failing us. The enormous wealth we pay for "health care" is not really making us more healthy. We live longer, work and produce - and consume more, only to fall victim to epidemics of modern chronic diseases such as heart disease, stroke, arthritis, diabetes, auto-immune diseases, Alzheimers, and "The Big C" - cancer.

Our air is being fouled and poisoned with tars, soots, asbestos and organic oils which cause lung cancer. Vinyl chloride, and pthalates from plastics are damaging our livers. We eat toxic dioxans and the lesser pesticides on our foods, which may also carry aflatoxins and nitrosamines, polycyclic aromatic hydrocarbons, and the ubiquitous benzopyrenes. Herbicides are acting like hormones in our bodies. Our DNA is unravelling in a chemical soup approved for our consumption by Health Canada, based on research submitted largely by the chemical, food and drug industries.

The naturopathic creed is not a backward march into prehistory.
We do stand proudly for some traditional values in dietetics and hygiene. If this is inconvenient for the consumer society and the drug based medical system, it is not intentional. People simply have the right to refuse to have noxious substances put into them. Life in Nature can be a hard road, but it has a way of keeping going.

We must be prudent to choose the level of medical care that is most appropriate because:
Cancer is not a benign or self-limiting disease.
It is unstable, dangerous, and unforgiving of poor choices.

CHARACTERISTICS OF CANCER CELLS

Cancer is a disorder of the control of growth of cells. Cancer cells grow faster than normal cells from the same tissue or organ.

Cells have the genetic code on their chromosomes, in the form of DNA. Each cell has about 2 meters of DNA, coiled incredibly tightly in a double spiral with links like steps on a ladder formed by 4 alkaline chemicals called *bases*. Using 4 letters (bases) arranged into 3 letter words (codons) the DNA library has all the information needed to create all the different cell shapes, sizes and products to form tissues, organs and the whole individual human being. Normal cells read only parts of the whole library, and become specialized or *differentiated* for a particular job in a particular place.

Cells should grow until they touch another cell, then stop - this is called *contact inhibition*. Cellular adhesion molecules (CAM) touching another cell results in a signal being sent from the cell's outer membrane surface to the DNA in the nucleus of the cell. It tells the DNA to stop growth of the cell, as it has reached its neighbour's property line.

Cells should have a limited lifespan, duplicating themselves a few dozen times. Repeated copying of the genetic information produces errors and missing bits in the DNA, so it begins to look like a bad photcopy. The aging normal cell removes a bit of the end of the chromosomes called a *telomere* everytime it is copied. When that telomere is gone, the cell cannot be copied, just like a videocassette with the little plastic tab removed cannot be recorded anymore. When the cell is old and has some errors that cannot be repaired, it will then quietly dissolve away in a natural process called apoptosis, to be replaced by a new cell.

Cancer cells develop from changes in the DNA called *mutations*.
Most mutations do not work out to be good for a cell's survival, but sometimes the cell gets lucky and finds a trick to grow relentlessly in an uncontrolled way, piling up into great masses. The cancer cells also become 'immortal' in the sense that they have no set lifespan. They can double and double and never throw the apoptosis switch to die. This means they make far more copies of their DNA than they were designed to, so the DNA becomes riddled with errors and abnormalities, making them unstable and bizarre acting. Tumor cells are unpredictable because they are genetically unstable and constantly evolving new genetic variations.

For those readers who would like a scientific explanation of the biology of cancer, here are some of the events at a molecular and cellular level that are necessary for cells to become malignant:

- Dysregulation results from DNA instability triggered by oxidative damage - over 10,000 oxidative hits per cell per day - causing non-lethal mutation. Free radicals of oxygen release lightning bolts of energy which break up the DNA. Healthy levels of antioxidants like vitamin A, C, E, selenium, and glutathione reduce the free radicals, and enzymes in the cell nucleus repair the damage if it is not too severe.

- Redox (reduction or oxidation) reactions occur when cells are exposed to excessive levels of trace minerals such as iron and copper. Redox agents produce dangerous free radicals and reactive oxygen species (ROS) which can activate or deactivate proteins - including genetic control proteins such as transcription factor p53, nuclear factor kappa B (NFkB) and activator protein 1 (AP-1). AP-1 is activated by hypoxia, a low oxygen level, which is seen in fast growing tumors which outstrip their blood supply.

- Inflammation reactions by the immune cells produce ROS, which increase mutation rates, DNA transcription (copying), and cell *growth factors*. These increase proliferation - the growth of more cancer cells. Cancer cells can counter-attack our immune cell ROS by producing immune suppressive factors such as cytokines IL-10, TGF-beta & prostaglandin PGE2.

- ROS also produce disulphide bonds between sulphur atoms as on cysteine moieties in DNA bases. This makes a chemical cross-link between DNA strands to form a *dimer*, rendering both strands unreadable. Repair of some DNA dimers is possible, but if too many accumulate, the cell will die. Antioxidants protect the DNA from these sulphur bonds gluing the pages of the genetic book shut. Antioxidants include vitamins C, E, carotenes, selenium, glutathione, alpha lipoic acid and grapeseed extract.

- Activation of *oncogenes* turns on changes in the DNA which lead a cell to become permanently transformed into the cancer lifestyle. Many appear to be retrovirus sequences which may have been spliced into our human ancestor's DNA by viral infection thousands of years ago. Other retroviruses may have entered with certain vaccinations extracted from animal cells infected with viruses.

- The human DNA genome library locked in the nucleus of every human cell, is now cluttered with millions of viral sequences: 1.3% is complete viral genomes - including oncogenes - which can trigger cancer directly. 10% of our genome consists of hundreds of thousands of copies of the viral promoter *Alu*, each only 280 base-pair sequences long. If these get turned on, all kinds of viruses lurking in the body, perhaps even lurking inside the cell's nucleus, can become active. An immune system overwhelmed by viruses cannot fight cancer.
15% of our genes code for the viral enzyme reverse transcriptase. This turns on viruses made of RNA, which we have lots of, including monkey RNA viruses from vaccinations, relatives of the HIV/AIDS retrovirus. We also may have DNA viruses such as SV40 from Salk polio virus grown on rhesus monkey kidney cells.

- Viruses can cause some cancers:
  - squamous cancers such as cervical carcinoma (HPV- human papilloma virus)
  - Burkitt's lymphoma, Hodgkin's Disease and nasopharyngeal carcinoma (EBV- Epstein-Barr virus)
  - Karposi's sarcoma (herpes virus).
  - Hepatocellular carcinoma / hepatoma (Hepatitis B or C virus)
  - T-cell leukemia and lymphoma (T-cell lymphotophic virus-1)
  - lymphoma, brain, bone and mesothelioma (SV-40 simian)

- Genetic expression becomes abnormal in many ways in a cancer cell. The cell may produce less than normal of growth inhibitors or may increase and facilitate DNA copying (transcription) factors. Overproduction of growth factors can also occur, such as transforming growth factor alpha (TGFa) which binds to epidermal growth factor receptors, and can transform the cell growth pattern and "immortalize" a cell when overexpressed.

- Transforming growth factor beta (TGF-b) is a potent immunosuppressor, making it harder for immune cells to find and kill cancer cells. TGF also induces angiogenesis, making blood vessels grow into the tumor to feed it oxygen and nutrients. TGF deregulates pericellular proteolysis - it allows cells to make enzymes which dissolve the protein barriers around it - which can allow the cancer cell to creep away and spread to new sites. Cancers which learn to produce more of this compound are much more dangerous.

- One DNA base can accept a methyl group - a carbon with a few hydrogens attached (-CH3) . When methylated, that part of the DNA cannot be opened, read and used. Reduced cytosine base methylation in cancer cells increases the rate of DNA transcription and therefore expression of most genes, including the bad ones. Fortunately dietary methyl group donors and antioxidants can increase methylation, reducing malignant gene over-expression. These include vitamins B12, B2, B6, folic acid, and betaine, all found in whole foods and vegetables. Folate is critical for the synthesis of s-adenosylmethionine (SAMe) which is the final methyl donor to DNA. Methylation defects produce excessive gene transcription. We can monitor serum homocysteine and urinary methylmalonic acid (MMA) as markers of this problem. Demethylation will unmask viral gene and oncogene sequences embedded in our DNA, which may be a critical step in the development of cancer . Also 'unsilenced' by demethylation are many growth promoter genes. These make existing cancers grow even faster.

- Growth factor receptors on the cell membranes may mutate and deliver continuous mitogenic (growth) signals, like a gas pedal that jams, putting growth on full throttle. Mitosis is another word for the doubling of the DNA and its separation and division into 2 new cells. Transmembrane receptors for growth factors, such as epidermal growth factor receptor (EGFR), have an extracellular binding region (on the outside of the cell) and an intercellular kinase (on the inside of the cell wall). Ligand binding (contact with its target molecule) results in homo- or hetero- dimer formation with activation of the associated tyrosine kinase inside the cell. This triggers several intracellular pathways, such as mitogen-activated protein kinase (MAPK) and AKT/P13K, which result in increased growth, resistance to apoptosis and increased angiogenesis. All of this means more cancer cell growth.

- Cell division is normally regulated by epidermal growth factor (EGF), platelet-derived growth factor (PDGF), transforming growth factor beta 1 (TGFB1) and insulin-like growth factor 1 (IGF-1). Normal signal transduction from the cell surface receptors to the nucleus occurs by way of phosphorylated tyrosine kinases (PTK). A receptor activated by its growth factor will make the PTK add fats on the inside of the cell. Lipid isoprenyloid tails on PTK's activate ras proteins which become trapped in their excitatory guanidine tri-phosphate-bound (GTP) forms. This activates cyclin-dependent kinases. Cyclins tell the cell to enter its cell cycle, its reproduction process. The cell copies itself and splits in two.

- Abnormal cell-to-cell communication at cell adhesion molecules (CAM) and gap junctions causes loss of contact inhibition, so the cells keep growing even after they bump up against another cell and should stop. This makes cells pile up into hard tumors - and still they grow! An independent cell is malignant, unable to act in the interest of the common good of the body network.

- The surface of cancer cells sends its nucleus "do not die" signals more than "do die" messages, so it never dies. When I grew human cells for research, we could only keep them going a few dozen generations of doubling, then they would expire. In a living person the cells also shut down after just a few dozen copies. No one can make a normal human cell live longer. However, we also grew
HeLa cells, which are human cervical squamous cancer cells from a woman named Helen Lane who had died of this disease in Baltimore, Maryland in 1951. Her cancer cells appear to be immortal. They grow incessantly, and never shut themselves off. All over the world, research labs have these and similar cancer cells which can be kept going indefinitely. Normal cells turn themselves off permanently when they accumulate errors from repeated copying. This gentle process is *apoptosis* or programmed cell death. Apoptosis should result in cells being quietly and safely removed and recycled.
Cancer cells can be made to undergo apoptosis if treated with natural agents!

- Cell cycle entry and progression results in cancer cell division and tumor growth. This step is normally regulated by Rb, Wt-1 and p53 tumor suppressor genes. p53 is known as the Guardian of the DNA because it arrests the cell cycle at the G1-S checkpoint, assesses for DNA damage, attempts to repair damage and mutations, and initiates cell suicide if it is unable to make repairs. The most dangerous and intractable cancers - melanoma, prostate, lung, bladder and colorectal cancers - have early occurrence of p53 mutations which reduce apoptotic removal of abnormal cells. Other cancers also can develop this problem, and so become more difficult to cure. Fortunately, sometimes the p53 can be encouraged to resume more normal levels of control over cell growth.
Natural agents supporting p53 activity can reverse the abnormal control of cell growth which is the very core of the cancer problem.

- Survival or anti-apoptotic signals arising from hormones, growth factors and cytokines may be altered by mutations affecting their cell surface receptors.

- Tumor necrosis factor (TNF) and *fas* gene protein ligands bind to plasma receptors to activate apoptosis initiator caspase enzymes, which then trigger "execution" caspases, which activate endonucleases and catabolic enzymes. This dissolves the damaged DNA and kills the cell.

- Reduced apoptosis in cancer cells increases malignancy - how dangerous a cancer is - by increasing cell survival and longevity.
  Old cancer cells accumulate DNA damage, DNA instability, and mutations. They get tougher to treat and are faster growing!

- The more undifferentiated a cell is, the more likely it will lose its sense of place and purpose, and lose the controls put on it by the specialized cells around it. It also means it can be less specific about the conditions under which it can live, so it will be better able to spread and grow in the wrong places. If a cell is completely dedifferentiated it is called anaplastic. If it is only partly dedifferentiated it is dysplastic. Natural agents which support cell differentiation can help a cancer cell remember how to behave appropriately, and reduce its survival in other tissues.

- How does any cell know what part of the huge library of DNA information it is expected to use? Cells have the whole library, but open up a small part by unmasking part of the DNA. Imagine a cell entering a library, opening up a book, studying it, using the information, and becoming trained to have a certain career.
  Just as an electrician studies electricity while a lawyer studies law, each cell uses part of the library. An eye cell acts like an eye cell and a stomach cell acts like a stomach cell because each makes different special enzymes from specific parts of the DNA. These enzymes make chemical reactions happen to give that cell what it needs for its specialized or 'differentiated' way of life. So how does it know what part to open up and read? By where it is in space relative to other cells, within electrical, magnetic and especially chemical gradients. The signals from its surrounding network vary by how far from the top, front or middle it is. Normal cells know where they are, and behave accordingly. In fact, if they are moved too far away they may fail to grow. Cancer cells becoming undifferentiated specialize in one thing only - growing fast and spreading to new places. They can open up all sorts of new parts of the DNA code, to adapt to new surroundings. They can also open up parts of the code to make chemicals which are toxic, or which allow other bad behaviour.

- Angiogenesis is the growth of new blood vessels to growing tissue. It happens in healing cuts and wounds and it happens for growing cancerous tumors. Arteries run into little capillaries which supply vital blood and nutrients to nearby cells. Angiogenesis is required for growth of a tumor past a very small size - 1 to 2 millimeters in diameter. This size tumor is undetectable, still safely localized at the *in situ* stage. New endothelial cells in the vascular buds secrete growth stimulating polypeptides such as IGF, Gm-CSF, PDGF and IL-1. Once a cancerous tumor has mastery over angiogenesis, it can grow large enough to kill the patient.

- Stressed cells produce heat shock proteins (HSP's) which prepare the cell for additional stress. Cancer cells can make HSP's to try to stay alive. For example, HSP's form a complex with mutant forms of p53 protein, produced by mutations on the p53 gene, and this complex disrupts normal mechanisms which would arrest the cancer cell growth cycle. Blocking HSP's will increase cancer cell death. Release of heat shock proteins into the circulation stimulates an immune response. This is one of the few things a cancer cell can do which will attract the attention of an immune cell. All too often the cancer cell looks normal to the immune cells, and goes unchecked until it is so deranged it cannot be stopped. Hyperthermia (heating) treatments may work in part by increasing immune system awareness of the cancer cells.

- We have 97% the same genes as a chimpanzee. We have 90% of the same genes as a corn plant. In fact only 3% of our genetic material in every one of our cells is actually needed to code for our unique human proteins! It is astonishing how much every living thing on the planet has in common at a genetic and biochemical level. This is the crux of why we believe remedies from the natural world are generally safer, because they have to be compatible with the same basic life processes.

SUMMARY

Tumor progression is characterized by progressive evolution of clones of cells with declining sensitivity to growth inhibition signals, evasion of apoptosis, sustained tumor-mediated angiogenesis, and an evolving ability to invade and metastasize.

As DNA monitoring and repair breaks down, and oncogenes are unmasked, the mutation rate of cells outstrips the genetic and immune controls. A cell must accumulate several peculiar biochemical skills before it can be a cancer. Many cells die trying, making fatal mutations or missing key steps. Those that do succeed in becoming cancerous continue to mutate and develop more and more ways to grow faster than their normal neighbours.

A million cells is the size of the head of a pin - undetectable, and so is called *occult cancer*, meaning "hidden". By a billion cells, it is the size of a small marble, and possibly detectable by touch or scans. This is called *clinical cancer* and it is as few as 30 doublings old. This mass weighs about 1 gram. After just 10 more doublings it can grow to 1 kilogram, which can often be fatal.

CARCINOGENESIS

There are 3 distinct phases in the growth of a tumor.

1. <u>Induction</u> - Genetic, viral, and environmental factors trigger malignant patterns of cell growth. Ultraviolet light and radiation causes DNA base fusion. ROS add oxygen compounds to the bases. Persistent oxidative stress and synergy with promoters such as hormones, phenols, and phorbol esters contribute to mutation and dedifferentiation. Chemical alkylating agents add methyl groups to the bases. Irreversible DNA damage or mutation occurs, especially to tumor suppressor genes Rb, CDK4, cyclin d and p16. Oncogenes turn on, DNA repair and apoptosis genes are turned off, and a cancer is born.

2. <u>Progression</u> - After loss of 2 or more suppressor genes and activation of several oncogenes there follows a period of growth of the transformed malignant cell clones. The environment must continue to support mutation and development of angiogenesis, invasion of adjacent tissues, immune evasion and other malignant characteristics. The descendants or clones of the original cancer cell change into a variety of mutants, so in fact there are several types of cancer within every large tumor.

3. <u>Proliferation</u> - 30 doublings produce 1 gram or about a billion cells, the threshold of detection, and in 10 more doublings produce 1 kilogram of tumor, which may be incompatible with life. Heterogeneous (mixed cell type) tumors are capable of rapid growth, invasion and metastasis. These are the hallmarks of cancer.

CANCER BY CELL TYPES

- Carcinomas - originate in epithelial tissue, and include squamous cell, transitional cell, basal cell and adenocarcinoma. These are the most common types of cancers, and the ones the immune system is most likely to miss detecting and responding to until quite late in the course of the disease. Dermal use of immune stimulants are always indicated.

- Sarcomas - arise in mesenchymal tissues such as muscles, skeleton, blood vessels, lymph vessels and reticular tissue; eg. osteosarcoma, myosarcoma, fibrosarcoma. Homotoxicology drainage remedies for the mesenchyme are always indicated.

- Lymphomas and leukemias - begin in lymphatic reticular tissue, a subset of mesenchyme stem cells from the bone marrow; includes Hodgkin's disease, lymphatic & myeloid leukemias. In Chinese medicine we look at the kidney and spleen to regulate blood building.

- Neuromas - develop in nerve tissue, and include glioblastoma multiforme, astrocytoma, neuroblastoma, meningioma, and pheochromocytoma. Dietary fats, fat-soluble toxins and antioxidants are often key issues.

- Other malignancies - hydatidiform mole, teratoma. As for all tumors, in Traditional Chinese Medicine a lump results from stagnant blood, which stopped moving due to deficiency of chi flow, arising from constrained liver chi.

Whatever the spot on the DNA or the cell surface or where in the body, cancer arises from living beyond the safe limits of cell chemistry. This incredible self-repairing organism can take a lot of abuse. It forgives a lot of exposures and it tolerates a lot of malnutrition.

Once cancer arises, the environment around the cell can be detoxified, the cells can be nourished, and the immune cells activated to create *healing conditions*.

Chapter Two -   CANCER AT THE ORGANISM LEVEL
It can take up to 20 years from the time the DNA damage reaches the point where the cell is permanently transformed into a lifestyle of uncontrolled growth to the point where it starts to harm organs and the whole person. Cancerous or malignant tumors are dangerous, toxic and parasitic. Cancer cells are out of touch with their neighbours and community, like dangerous renegades. There is always to some extent an immune system failure where cancer persists.

SURVIVAL RATES

- The most generally useful measure is 5 year survival disease-free. This allows comparison of the effects of different treatments. Often a patient who lives 5 years without a sign of the original cancer is truly cured. However, such survival statistics do include people who will die of their cancer due to delayed re-occurrences, who have enjoyed a long remission or pause in the disease.

- Individual survival is NOT predictable with much accuracy! No one can really say with certainty how long a patient will survive. All we can predict is the average survival time, based on present standards of care. There is naturally always hope of increased life and quality of life with natural medicine support to enhance regular medical care.

- There is always hope of a miracle by Divine intervention, luck, or whatever you can find to believe in. Do not ever give up! A wise man once said "Fear is faith in evil". Believe in good and the grace of peace will come to you.

- Quality of life may be severely and irrevocably diminished by medical oncology. Natural and drug adjuncts are supportive therapies which reduce harm and increase the potential for successful treatment outcomes.

- Allopathic medicine has reasonable success treating leukemias and lymphomas, and skin cancers. Localized *in situ* cancers are typically 50 to 80% curable. Spread into regional lymph nodes is a sign of aggressive disease with a poorer prognosis, often less than 50% survival. Distant metastases are rarely curable but effective palliation can give 5 to 20% 5 year survival. For the most common and majority of cancers there has been no significant change in survival rates in modern times. Cancer remains a traumatic disease with a generally unfavorable outcome.

GRADING

- Grading is done by a pathologist looking at cancer cells stained to make them visible under a microscope. The severity of the cancerous changes is given based on the degree of differentiation of tumor cells, and on the number of mitoses with highly condensed chromatin figures - the number of cells caught in the act of making an extra copy of their DNA. More differentiation means more normal specialization for a particular job. More mitoses mean it is growing fast.

- Grades I to IV are usually assigned, a higher number meaning increasing anaplasia - loss of recognizable differentiation. Anaplastic cells are wild and dangerous.

- Histology (cell architecture) does not necessarily determine the clinical behaviour of the tumor. In other words, you cannot see through a microscope exactly how the cancer will behave in the body, so grading is only part of the information needed to decide on therapies.

The practice of medicine is informed by data, but clinical judgement is based on the subjective elements of perception, experience and belief.

STAGING

Staging is based on the key characteristics of cancer:
> proliferation - uncontrolled growth
> invasion - pushing into neighbors
> metastasis - spread to other organs

- Size of the primary lesion (T)
- Extent of spread into regional lymph nodes (N)
- Blood-borne metastases to distant locations (M)

This is clinically critical information in selecting therapies and making a prognosis - an estimate of the outcome of the disease.

APOPTOSIS

This is the ideal way to remove problem cells or cells no longer needed in the body. It is a "Magic Bullet" which gently takes out unwanted cells with no harm to any other cell. It is the future of curing cancer in a humane way.

- "Programmed cell death" or cell suicide is rapid, orderly, and removes individual cells. Nearby cells are not harmed. This is a normal part of the growth and maintenence of healthy tissues.

- Apoptosis is triggered by a preponderance of "do die" signals over "do not die" signals sent to the DNA. This is a dynamic balance, like yin and yang, both are always present, but the overall balance determines the net outcome.

- Energy-dependent, apoptosis requires the basic energy molecule adenosine tri-phosphate (ATP), usually made by burning sugars.

- Cells undergoing apoptosis show cell shrinkage, chromatin condensation making the DNA visible in the nucleus, surface blebbing (bubbles), and fragmentation into apoptotic bodies -membrane-bound bits of the stuff from inside the cells - the cytoplasm (liquid) and organelles (structures).

- Phagocytosis or the eating and digestion of whole cells or apoptotic bodies (cell fragments) is carried out by parenchymal cells in tissues or macrophage immune cells. Digestion in their enzyme-filled organelles called lysozomes is rapid.

- No inflammation or immunological reactions are created. There is no release of iron or other metallic ions that can cause oxidative stress.

- Apoptosis promoters from Nature include quercitin, curcumin, betulinic acid, caffeine, genestein, berberine, vitamin E succinate, glutathione, N-acetyl cysteine and mistletoe (viscum) lectins. These are antioxidants and bioflavenoids from apples, onions, tumeric, soybeans, coffee and other food grade plants as well as herbs or botanical medicines such as mistletoe.

INVASION

Cancer does little harm growing into a simple lump. It could be just removed by a surgeon and tossed away if that were all it could do. Because cancer cells stop communicating normally with their neighbours, they can push past them and spread into surrounding structures, and beyond. This is where the tumor becomes a serious problem.

- Cancer cells lose contact inhibition, primarily through changes to cell adhesion molecules and gap junction proteins.

- Cancer cells may over-produce proteolytic enzymes, which dissolve the extracellular matrix (ECM) which binds cells together.
    Growing tumors can then progressively infiltrate through the basement membrane that normally forms a boundary for a tissue. This is like a prisoner digging an escape tunnel out of where it supposed to stay – now it can get loose and do harm.

- Single tumor cells or clusters are shed from tumors as normal cell-to-cell adherins are down-regulated, by mechanical and hydrostatic pressure, central necrosis, and by proteolytic enzymes. Adherins are like a glue or clamp that keeps cells stuck to each other.

- Receptors on the tumor cells learn to adhere to laminin and fibronectin proteins in the extracellular matrix (ECM) rather than just to other cells.   The matrix fills in the space between cells, and learning to ride the matrix gives cancer cells a highway out of town.

- Motility can involve creeping along ECM protein fibres as they are pulled into the cancer cell for digestion. Its food becomes a path of escape.

- Collagens, glycoproteins and proteoglycans in the ECM are enzymatically digested. Breakdown products of the ECM are growth-promoting, angiogenic, and chemotactic. These increase tumor growth and movement in a vicious cycle.

- Penetration into blood vessels, lymphatic channels and body cavities allows the opportunity to spread.

METASTASIS

Metastases or *mets* are the most dangerous aspect of a malignant tumor. Successful colonization of a distant part of the body with cancer usually means much poorer chance of recovery.

- A metastasis is a discontinuous secondary tumor made of one of the cell types found in the original tumor. For example, a metastasis of breast cancer to the brain means the "brain met" is still made of breast cancer cells, not brain cells.

- Generally a "met" will be clones or descendants of cancer cells which are particularly mutated to be aggressive, rapidly growing, treatment-resistant, and anaplastic.

- Primary sites of metastases and screening methods:
    bone - radioisotope bone scans
    liver - elevated LDH enzyme in serum
    lung - CT scan or cytology from bronchoscopy
    brain - CT or MRI scan

- Disseminated metastases must evade immune surveillance. Immune cells may be killing millions of these wandering cells daily. It is likely that all tumors shed millions of cells daily, but it is actually quite rare for such wanderers to survive.

- A metastatic cell must then adhere to endothelial cells lining the blood vessels in the target organ. Insulin-like growth factors I and II are chemoattractants for metastases. The cell will stop and attach where it "smells" this chemical. These are high when the diet is rich in sugars and simple carbohydrates.

- Metastases must then extravasate, or leave the blood vessel through the basement membrane of the endothelium lining to enter the new tissue.

- Metastases only grow significantly if they can stimulate angiogenesis or new blood vessel growth into their new home.

- Natural anti-metastatics include fractionated or modified citrus pectin (MCP), larch arabinogalactan, aloe vera juice, eicosapentanoic fatty acid (EPA), conjugated linoleic acid (CLA), bromelain and heparin.

ANGIOGENESIS

Cancers by definition are growing faster than the normal cells of their type. They can have 30 to 40 times normal basal metabolic rate. Therefore they must have even greater than normal amounts of oxygen and nutrients, requiring a blood supply greater than normal for that tissue. New blood vessels sprout and extend into tissues that are low in oxygen. These *hypoxic* cells release chemicals which trigger angiogenesis.

- Formation of new blood supply to hypoxic cells is a normal part of wound healing. Cancer is "the wound that will not heal".

- Angiogenesis is necessary for tumor growth beyond a few millimeters in diameter.

- Redundant mechanisms drive the induction of blood vessel growth. This duplication and layering of controls makes it a complex business to alter angiogenesis.

- "Angiogenesis occurs in and produces an environment steeped in growth factors" which can severely reduce apoptosis in tumors at the same time as it feeds rapid growth.

- Capillary basement membranes dissolve, a bud grows, and elongates along a collagen scaffolding into the hypoxic zone.

- In tumors the vessel loops formed tend to be chaotic, thin-walled, and leaky, increasing risk of spread of cancer cells into the general circulation. The fluid build-up (edema) leaking into the tumor increases the osmotic fluid pressure in the tumor, which can squeeze off blood flow, and trigger a new round of hypoxia and angiogenesis.

- The primary angiogenic triggering compound is vascular endothelial growth factor (VEGF) a highly conserved heparin-binding glycoprotein which induces endothelial cell mitogenesis and migration, increases vascular permeability and vasodilation, induces proteinases which remodel the extracellular matrix, inhibits antigen-presenting dendritic immune cells, and inhibits endothelial cell apoptosis. VEGF expression is regulated by hypoxia, and mediated by 3 distinct cell surface receptors as well as 2 co-receptors. The tyrosine kinase domain Flk-1 and Flt-1 play a critical role in tumor angiogenesis, and have been the targets of research with humanized recombinant monoclonal antibodies.

- Also important in angiogenesis are basic fibroblast growth factor (bFGF) and various growth regulator compounds including insulin, tumor necrosis factor (TNF), lactic acid, histamine, prostaglandins and fibrin.

- Copper is an essential mineral for many angiogenesis promoters. It is proven to reduce circulating levels of vasculoendothelial growth factor (VEGF), fibroblast growth factor 2 (FGF2), and interleukins 6 and 8 (IL-6, IL-8). Angiogenesis promoters angiotropin, angiogenin, and cysteine-rich proteins are copper dependent. Copper can be removed by chelating with tetrathiomolybdate (TM) Treatment for three months will usually reduce copper to about 20% of baseline levels, which will often arrest tumor growth. The TM is given with food to bind the copper in the food, and also given between meals to bind-up blood copper. As copper is involved in heme synthesis and red blood cell proliferation, a side effect can be anemia and mild leukopenia, reversible on easing up the therapy. A low copper diet and zinc supplements can keep levels steady. Monitor ceruloplasmin in the blood, a protein made in the liver, incorporating 6 to 7 atoms of copper, which transports iron from the liver to the bone marrow. Use purified water if your home has copper pipes. Anti-copper therapies like TM only inhibit small tumors, larger ones tend to escape its effect via alternative angiogenic pathways.

- Ischemia (hypoxia caused by reduced blood flow) and inflammation activate an endogenous cholinergic angiogenic pathway. This pathway is independent of VEGF and bFGF, and is stimulated by nicotine. Tobacco products cause blood vessels to constrict for hours after exposure, and this adds insult to injury.

- Surgery is never done on a tumor if there is evidence of smaller metastatic lesions. Removing the original or 'mother' tumor can cause the remaining tumors to grow very quickly. As long as the mother is left in place, it puts out signals which slow angiogenesis in the others, keeping them smaller.

- Antiangiogenesis agents induce tumor stasis, not tumor regression - they stop the cancer from growing bigger but may not get rid of the cancer.

- Natural anti-angiogenic compounds include catechin, EGCG from green tea, curcumin, vitamins A, D & E, mushroom shikonin, soy genestein isoflavone, and shark liver oil. Use COX II inhibitors. Consider sodium chromoglycolate.

IMMUNE EVASION

- Healthy adults may produce 500 to 1000 new cancer cells daily. Dr. Kobayashi screened asymptomatic adults and estimates only 1 in 1000 is completely cancer free. 70.6% had precancerous cells, about 25% had pre-clinical cancers, and about 5% had undiagnosed clinical cancer - tumors over 1 gram.

- NK cells and apoptosis remove most cancers as they arise. Uncontrolled cells can produce diagnosable malignant disease in about 5 to 20 years.

- Natural killer (NK) cells are large lymphocytes specialized to kill viral infected, solid tumor or leukemic cells. Up to 15% of total lymphocytes are NK's. Exercise increases NK cell counts.

- Remedies which increase NK activity, as measured from bioactivity assays from the patient's blood, have no reliable significant clinical effect on cancer outcomes. Beware of claims that a product will cure cancer based only on its impact on NK cell number or activity. Natural Killer cells can only kill cancer when other immune cells such as macrophages support them or at least refrain from blocking them.

- Tumors may shed up to 3 to 4 million cancer cells per gram of tumor per day, yet successful metastasis is relatively rare.

- The immune system can be overwhelmed by large tumors or metastases, especially cell clusters. These may arise from a traumatic blow to a tumor, cutting into the cancer in surgery, etc.

- Cancers develop techniques to block the processing of their antigens, proteins which tell the immune cells they are not behaving normally. Tumor cells evade recognition by modulation of surface proteins, antigenic degradation, absorption or shedding, shedding of TNF receptors, and induced immunosuppression. Thymus activated immune T-cells can destroy tumor cells only with adequate tumor antigen presentation by macrophages and dendritic cells. Naturopathic physicians always use thymus for cancer care: glandulars, extracts, peptides or homeopathics. I like Dolisos homeopathic *Thymuline.*

- Viral-associated cancers such as cervical squamous cell carcinoma, Karposi's sarcoma, Burkitt's lymphoma and T-cell leukemias and lymphomas are also associated with immune suppression such as in AIDS/HIV/ARC. (Acquired Imunnodeficiency Syndrome, Human immunodeficiency Virus, and AIDS Related Complex)

- Melanoma, lymphoma and renal (kidney) cell carcinoma express tumor-associated antigens, and have been known to respond to immune modulating therapies such as monoclonal antibodies and vaccines. Other cancer types are less likely to respond to immune therapies.

- Current active immunotherapy techniques are still crude and expensive, but progress is being made identifying antigenic targets (molecular profiling of cancer cells), overcoming negative regulatory mechanisms, and making antibodies with attached toxins, radionuclides, and light-activated poisons. About 400 monoclonal antibodies are in clinical trials.

See Chapter Seven - Immune Therapies - p. 128

INFLAMMATION & CANCER SURVIVAL

Inflammation results in the release of *cytokines* - leukotrienes, eicosanoids, prostaglandins. Cytokines are chemical signals which trigger normal cells to grow to repair and replace tissues as they age or those damaged by infection or trauma. Cytokines can also trigger cancer cells to grow. Dr. Pooh Bear calls this
"Not A Very Good Thing".

High levels of inflammation correspond to the Chinese medicine concept of 'fire poison' or 'heat toxin'. When this is present, the patient is in great danger, and uncontrolled, death often follows soon. This is becoming recognized in Western medicine. The measurement of blood markers for systemic inflammation such as serum C-reactive protein (CRP) is now being used to assess survival prognosis. Note that high levels correspond to increase risk of death from cancer, heart disease and many other risks. The hazard rating from all causes increases about three fold with every ten fold increase in CRP.

History of chronic use of non-steroidal anti-inflammatory drugs (NSAIDS) is associated with up to 50% reduced risk of breast and colon cancers. These drugs block cytokines sucha as prostaglandins. Prostaglandins are eicosanoids made from dietary polyunsaturated fatty acids by the action of cyclooxygenase enzymes (COX 1 and 2). COX-2 makes series-2 prostaglandins PGE-2 and PGE-2a which are hormone-like compounds acting locally to produce pain, inflammation and swelling. COX-2 and its product PGE-2 contribute to tumor viability and progression by increasing cell proliferation, inhibiting apoptosis, increasing angiogenesis, increasing invasiveness, increasing metastasis, and by immunosuppression.

COX-2 is stimulated by tumor promoters, growth factors, angiogenesis factors such as VEGF, and cytokines. Inducers include oncogenes ras and scr, ultraviolet radiation, hypoxia, IL-1, EGF, TGF-b, TNF-a and benzo(a)pyrene.

COX-2 mRNA and protein overexpression is found in epithelial tumors, colorectal cancer tissue, gastric, pancreatic and many other carcinoma biopsy samples, and in brain gliomas. Increased expression is signifigantly correlated with unfavorable clinico-pathological characteristics such as worse tumor size, stage, de-differentiation, lymph node involvement, vascularization (angiogenesis) and metastases.

Low COX-2 expression and receptor levels strongly correlate with extended survival in cervical carcinoma - 75% 5 year survival for patients with low values versus 35% 5 year survival for those with high levels.

The hormones progesterone and estradiol estrogen up-regulate COX activity. Healthy bodies produce these hormones, but they are also taken as drugs, and in our food from use in farm animals. Many agricultural pesticides, herbicides and chemical fertilizers mimic estrogens when they enter the human body. These chemicals which act like hormones even though they are not intended to, are called 'xenobiotics'. Xeno means foreign, man-made substances used for convenience, which turn on us and poison us.

COX-2 is linked to aromatase gene expression. PGE-2 activates aromatase to increase biosynthesis of estrogen in fat cells. This can produce a vicious cycle of estrogen dysregulation in breast cancer. Blocking the HER-2/neu signaling reduces COX-2 expression.

COX-2 up-regulates metallo-proteinases such as MMP-2 which increase tumor cell migration and invasion. Inflammation makes cancer spread.

Tumor derived PGE-2 promotes the production of the potent immunosuppressive cytokine IL-10 by lymphocytes and macrophages, while simultaneously inhibiting IL-2 production, a cytokine which dampens inflammation. PGE-2 also inhibits natural killer cells and lymphokine-activated killer cells.

Lipoxygenase (LOX) enzymes create inflammation, pain, vasoconstriction and thrombosis promoting compounds from arachidonic acid (AA). These include hydroxyeicosatetraenoic acids 5-HETE, 12-HETE and 15-HETE. A third pathway produces 12-HETE and 16-HETE directly using cytochrome p-450.

5 and 12-HETE and LOX product LTB4 are longer acting than COX products, strongly stimulate cancer cell growth and progression, and inhibit apoptosis. 12-HETE is associated with reduced cell adhesion, invasion and metastasis, and correlates with advanced stage and poor differentiation.

Hyperinsulinemia increases PGE-2 synthesis from dihomo-gammalinolenic acid (DGLA). Another good reason to limit sugar and refined foods in the diet!

Dietary measures to limit inflammatory eicosanoids -

- Restrict arachidonic acid rich foods – meat, dairy, poultry - a vegan diet does help, if correctly constructed.
- Reduce refined carbohydrates - processed starches, simple sugars and alcohol
- Eliminate hydrogenated fats and trans fatty acids - margarine, shortening and lard.
- Reduce intake of omega 6 plant oils - especially corn oil and corn-silage fed animal foods.
- Increase omega 3 oils from nuts, seeds, fish and sea mammals, and grass-fed land animals.
- Ingest adequate zinc, magnesium, vitamins A, B3 and B6, C and E.
- Botanical LOX inhibitors include green-lipped muscle extract, boswellia and scutellaria.
- Quercitin, curcumin and EPA marine oils inhibit both LOX and COX.
- Other COX-2 inhibitors are green tea EGCG, bromelain, licorice, grapeseed proanthocyanidin and garlic.

DIAGNOSIS

Biopsy and histological evaluation are the only way to confirm cancer. It is unethical to offer to treat as cancer a case not medically confirmed, nor can one claim a cure until the positive test results are reversed.

- Cytology is a method of looking at loose cells taken off tumors or from around them. Pap smears, washings or brushings during endoscopies, and needle aspiration are alternatives to removing the primary tumor for evaluation.

- Supported by physical exam, scans, X-ray imaging, hormones, antigens, antibodies, neurological findings, tumor markers and tumor specific scans.

TUMOR MARKERS

Cancer cells are so abnormal in so many ways, it is likely they will make and leak abnormal chemicals which we may detect in the blood. For generations now, researchers have noticed the striking similarity between cells growing as a cancer and the early cells growing in the trophoblast - the early embryo stage where our lives begin. Many cancers make chemicals that should not be seen in a person who is not pregnant or not a fetus.

Tumors often produce characteristic metabolites, antigens & hormones which are measurable in the blood by radio-immunoassays. Rarely is a single tumor marker test sensitive or accurate enough to be diagnostic, or even an effective screening method for early warning of the onset or return of a cancer. However, some attempts have been made to use panels of several of these tests for early detection, such as the Kobayashi panel of ten markers. This idea deserves further study.

Tumor markers are being used, with some caution, to guide diagnosis, prognosis, the initial therapeutic strategy and changes in therapeutics. They tend to fall if treatment response is good, and rise if the cancer is reoccurring. While they imply a cetain level of 'tumor burden', the amount produced by a cancer can vary, so a doubling of the level of tumor marker doesn't necessarily mean twice as many cancer cells are present. We like to see these numbers low or zero, but people can survive well with high numbers too. Your physician may choose to not tell you these numbers, as they can cause needless concern. What you need to hear most is that the physician is monitoring you and providing definitive, rational and comprehensive care.

Carcinoembryonic antigen (CEA) - non-specific, this chemical indicates undifferentiated cells are present, similar to those found in an embryo, where the cells are not yet committed to being a certain tissue. CEA can be raised in benign conditions and is not sensitive in early malignancy. Elevated in 20 to 70% of cancer patients depending on tumor site and stage. For example levels should fall to zero after complete resection of colon cancer, rising levels tend to suggest regrowth, and high levels are associated with a poorer prognosis.

Prostate specific antigen (PSA) - prostate cancer screening tool, rate of doubling is a signifigant indicator of tumor aggressiveness.

CA 125 - rising levels can indicate relapse and level of tumor burden in breast cancer. The CA stands for carbohydrate antigen.

Human chorionic gonadotrphin beta subunit (b-HCG) - is useful in germ cell tumors such as testicular cancer to monitor effect of treatment and reveal relapses. Home pregnancy tests detect this hormone.

Alpha-fetoprotein (AFP) - should not occur except in fetal blood, indicates hepatoma (up in 72% of cases), pancreatic (23%), gastric (18%) or germ cell tumors (75% of nonseminomatous testicular tumors). Post-therapy return to normal levels usually correlates with effective therapy.

Lactate dehydrogenase (LDH) - fast growing tumors in high S-phase outstrip their blood supply and become anaerobic, producing toxic lactic acid. LDH monitors cell death in oxygen starved tumors, and is also a marker for *tumor lysis* (break-up). It is raised in liver disease and blood hemolysis.

TUMOR MARKER BY ORGAN OR CELL TYPE

Breast - CEA, CA 15-3, CA 125, CA 549, CA M26, CA M29, CA 27.29, MCA, PSA, isoferritin, tissue polypeptide antigen (TPA), mammary tumor-associated glycoprotein, and kappa casein.

Prostate - prostate specific antigen (PSA), standard, ultrasensitive or free PSA, and prostatic acid phosphatase (PAP)

Gastro-intestinal - kappa casein

Stomach - fetal sulfoglycoprotein antigen

Liver - AFP, CEA; Liver mets - alkaline phosphatase, 5'-nucleotidase, glycolytic enzymes

Pancreas - CEA, TPA, pancreatic oncofetal antigen

Colon - CEA, TPA

Lung - small cell - NSE, CK-BB; CEA, TPA

Bone - alkaline phosphatase

Thyroid - calcitonin, thyroglobulin

Ovary - CEA, CA 125, galactosyl transferase

Testes - (germ cell) AFP, beta-chorionic gonadotrophin (b-HCG), LDH, placental-like AP

Leukemia - b2-microglobulin, isoferritin

Lymphoma - b2-microglobulin, monoclonal immunoglobulins; Epstein-Barr viral antibodies in Burkitt's lymphoma

Myeloma - Bence-Jones protein immunoglobulins, monoclonal immunoglobulins

Neuroblastoma - VMA, NSE, catecholamines; CNS - b2 microglobulin

Nasopharyngeal - Epstein-Barr viral antibodies

C.A.U.T.I.O.N. - Cancer Society 7 Cardinal Warning Signs of Cancer
- C hange in bowel or bladder habits
- A sore that does not heal
- U nusual bleeding or discharge
- T hickening or extension of a lump
- I ndigestion or difficulty swallowing
- O bvious change in a wart or mole
- N agging cough or hoarseness

Investigate these, sudden weight loss, or any disturbing health change. It may be alarming, but get an early diagnosis.

Chapter Three - MEDICAL TREATMENT SURVIVAL STRATEGIES

SURGERY

Surgery is the medical art of removing the patient from the disease.
It is generally a good idea to reduce the *tumor burden*. Less cancer cells can mean less medication to achieve cancer control.

- Exploratory, curative resection, palliation, reconstructive, catheterization - to stop hemorrhages, correct obstructions, and stop pain.

- Resectability depends on location, extent, fixation (what it is attached to), and spread to contiguous (nearby) or distant sites.

- The high risk surgical patient is malnourished, with unplanned loss of over 10 % of body weight, or serum albumen protein measuring under 3.5 gm/dl.

- Wide excision means cutting out a piece much bigger than the tumor. Due to the invasive tendency, there may be invisible penetration out from the borders of a tumor, so a surgeon tries to get *clean margins* by cutting beyond the visible tumor. The pathologist will check the boundary area under a microscope to confirm all cancer cells have been safely removed, plus a bit more for safety sake.

- Potential seeding or release of tumor mets by the handling of the tumor in surgery is still controversial. Some argue that this is not important, as the body deals with shed cells all the time. It is not ethical to suggest this risk exceeds the benefits of cancer surgery. While not well tested in human trials, modified citrus pectin and related products show great promise in animal studies to reduce this risk to nearly zero. In my practice, this product has never failed to perform!

- There may be de-inhibition of angiogenesis in mets when the "mother" or primary tumor is removed. Occassionally cancer "explodes" after surgery, as hidden mets suddenly grow wildly.

- Major surgery results in significant immunosuppression, which may increase metastatic spread, as well as the risk of infection.

PRE-OP PROTOCOL

1. Reduce metastasis risk with modified citrus pectin (MCP) 1 Tblsp. twice daily. Modified or fractionated citrus pectin, and larch arabinoglycans, work like putting flour on Scotch tape - mets can't stick to their new home, and if they are not attached to something they can't divide and grow.

2. Avoid for a week all herbs which interact with sedatives and anaesthetics: St. John's Wort *Hypericum perforatum*; valerian root - *Valeriana officinalis*; kava kava *Piper methysticum*. Also avoid natural medicines which can cause bleeding problems: EPA fish oils; garlic *Allium sativa*; gingko leaf *Gingko biloba*; ginseng root *Panax ginseng* or *Panax cinquefolium*; bromelain; vitamin K.

3. Surgery mix - 6C potency homeopathics *Hypericum*, *Staphysagria* and *Arnica* – this formula was given to me by Dr. Andre Saine, ND, a great homeopath. He told me patients will come back and say their surgeon told them "I've never seen anyone heal so fast" and that is exactly what has happened in many cases. The Hypericum treats nerve injury and pain, the Arnica helps relieve trauma, edema, inflammation, and the Staphysagria deals with the injury at an emotional and mental level.

4. Test for tumor markers before surgery, to establish a baseline for what that cancer produces when it is a certain size. Ideally, the marker will drop to zero after surgery, and then any rise will signal that the cancer may be returning.

5. Good nutrition: vitamin C - 2,000mg, zinc citrate - 60 mg; vitamin A -10,000 IU twice daily; high protein - which might include a whey powder supplement 1 ounce (30 grams) twice daily. It is very risky to operate when protein status is impaired - this was the cause of my father's death by surgical misadventure.

Start wound healing support 2 weeks pre-op.

POST-OP PROTOCOL

1. Reduce blood clot risk with 3,200 MCU strength Bromelain - 500 mg. 2 to 4 times daily away from protein foods; curcumin 500 mg. 3 times daily; EPA oils 2 to 4 grams daily with food, and physical activity.

2. Prevent adhesions and excessive scarring with catechins 500 mg. 3 times daily, gotu kola *Centella asiatica* yielding 50 to 100 mg of triterpenic acids, and vitamin E - 400 to 1,200 I.U. daily with food.

3. Support wound healing with zinc citrate - 50 to 60 mg twice daily with food; vitamin A - 50,000 I.U. daily; and vitamin C - 1000 mg. 3 times daily.

4. Probiotics are good bowel bacteria, essential to good health, and often diminished by stress and antibiotics. Take a capsule of enteric coated mixed bowel bacteria 2 to 3 times daily away from food, for up to 2 months.

5. Continue MCP at 12 grams or 2 tablespoons daily for up to 6 months. It is very sticky, so use a blender to put into juice.

6. Proteolytic enzymes reduce inflammation and swelling, prevent clots and prevent and treat venous thrombophlebitis. At the same time these enzymes can inhibit metastatic spread of cancer cells, inhibit angiogenesis to tumors, activate immune production of interferons against viruses, and help immune cells detect cancer.

7. Ferdinand Sauerbrach, a thoracic surgeon, has demonstrated improved surgical wound healing and increased resistance to infection with a salt-restricted diet.

8. Remember surgery is very immunosuppressive. This is the time for homeopathic, nutritional and herbal support for the immune system - for example, *Engystol*, *Thymuline*, vitamin A, vitamin C, zinc citrate, echinacea, cat's claw, and Reishi mushrooms.

9. A positive attitude and having friends pray for your recovery appears to make a real difference in outcome - less pain, less complications, faster healing, etc. Love really is the answer.

RADIATION

Ionizing radiation is a standard treatment for cancer, despite significant risks, side-effects, and about 1/3 of cases failing to achieve good local control of tumors. You may be shocked how little scientific evidence there is for survival benefits from many applications of radiotherapy. Here is a primer on radiotherapy:

- Releases a large amount of energy in a small, localized volume along the beam line (linear energy transfer or LET)

- Electromagnetic energies such as X-ray, gamma ray, or ultraviolet light produce indirect ionized particles of high energy and excited atoms with electrons in higher orbits, which are more chemically reactive. This creates havoc in our life chemistries.

- High speed sub-atomic particles - electrons, protons, neutrons, pi mesons. If they have over 10 electron volts of energy —they can produce direct ionization by ejecting electrons from atoms, which then break covalent chemical bonds, produce free radicals of oxygen (ROS), and secondary particle cascades. The large particles have a short range that is dependent on their initial kinetic energy or velocity.

- Ionizing radiation usually forms hydroxyl radicals [*OH) in water inside cells, which break strands of DNA, the genetic code. If both strands are broken, and go unrepaired, the cell will die. However, if one strand remains unrepaired, the cell survives, but in an altered form. Thus radiation can kill cancer cells, and cause normal cells to develop into cancer.

- DNA is a critical target - base damage and formation of dimers or bonds between strands are cytotoxic - the cell must repair or die.

- External beams such as X-ray devices, gamma ray "cobalt bomb", linear electron megavoltage accelerators (Lineacs) and the 'gamma knife' units bombard the body from the outside, so much of the energy gets absorbs into overlying tissues and doesn't reach the tumor. This is like sunlight going into water, it is absorbed near the surface and so can't get too deep.

- Implants such as rapid cesium pellet brachytherapy use high dose radioactive substances placed near a cancer to deliver a very high local dose. Many of these isotopes release high energy particles with large mass which cannot penetrate too far into healthy structures around the tumor.

- Rapidly dividing cells are most susceptible: cancers, small lymphocytes, bone marrow, vascular endothelium, gastrointestinal endothelium & hair follicles. That is why radiation kills cancer but also makes the hair fall out and the gut to be disturbed by sores, vomiting and diarrhea.

- Mitotic (doubling) delay at G2 in the cell cycle is proportional to the radiation dose, prolonging the generation time, producing non-dividing cells, chromosome aberrations, giant cells and cell death.

- Radiation is oncogenic, causing normal cells to become cancerous, with up to a 20 year induction phase. Decades after treatment there is a 6 times increased risk of a new solid tumor from radiotherapy for Hodgkin's disease, 4 to 5 times increased risk of esophageal cancer after radiotherapy of breast cancer, and increased occurrence of leukemia, breast, thyroid, lung and GI cancers after radiation exposure.

- Sclerosis or scarring and contraction of vascular endothelium (the lining of blood vessels) is slowly progressive, leading to endarteritis (inflamed lining), fibrosis & thrombus (clot) formation. Radiation to the heart is associated with increased risk of coronary artery disease. This scarring goes on relentlessly for years after the therapy. Given enough time, it will always degrade the ability of the tissue to heal.

- 1/3 local failure rate is mostly due to the hypoxic cell problem - 2.5 to 3 times higher doses are needed for the same biological effect in low oxygen parts of tumors than are used for fully oxygenated cells. Radiated oxygen and water produce reactive oxygen species (ROS). The most common from O_2 is the hydroxyl radical (OH^*) which typically causes single strand DNA breaks. Without oxygen the radiation energy does not get transformed into chemical energy which is what actually damages the cancer cell. My research area for several years at the British Columbia Cancer Research Foundation Medical Biophysics Unit was on this "hypoxic cell problem". We looked at new drugs and new radiation sources that would kill the cells living on the edge of survival in oxygen-deprived parts of a tumor.

If you have been given radiation therapy once, you may only receive it again if the total dose accumulated will be under 7,000 to 8,000 CentiGrays, as more is usually fatal.

It is interesting to note that children are given Carbogene gas to breathe before radiation therapy to make their tumors more sensitive to the therapy. This is 80% oxygen (O2) mixed with 20% carbon dioxide (CO2). Normal air is 21% oxygen and the rest is mostly nitrogen (N2).

I am frequently asked about hyperbaric oxygen therapy and cancer. Using 100% oxygen under pressure certainly delivers a massive dose of oxygen. We know it cures 'the Bends' in divers, but will it help to kill cancer? Well, the oxygen does increase chemical damage and cancer cell death from radiation. In early experiments adult patients combining radiation and hyperbaric oxygen often died immediately from the combination. It quickly went out of fashion. Still, some persist in suggesting it for general cancer care. Oxygen in really high doses does increase immune activity against cancer cells. However, it increases blood vessel growth into the tumor too. The net effect is neither good nor bad. I simply do not recommend it as an ethical cancer treatment. If hyperbaric therapy is needed for another life-threatening condition in a patient who has or may have cancer, I would not hesitate to use it.

A novel idea in contemporary radiation care is photodynamic therapy with ionized oxygen. Light of a specific wavelength is used to activate the ionically charged oxygen at the tumor only.

In all forms of cancer therapy it is important to support the clearance from the body of damaged cells and their debris. This means giving antioxidants, liver support, and help for the circulating and the reticulo-endothelial immmune system, which digest bad cells. Toxic therapies like radiation kill patients directly and indirectly, and often render them so debilitated they cannot then respond to complementary and alternative natural therapies. Integrating both orthodox and natural adjuncts (supports) helps keep the options open by protecting a reserve of vitality.

Be proactive, as all doses of radiation cause injury, though the symptoms may only appear much later on.

GENERAL RADIATION PROTECTANTS

Dr. Andrew Weil, M.D. states in his book *Spontaneous Healing*: "Remember that radiation and chemotherapy are themselves mutagenic and carcinogenic" and "In general, radiation is safer than chemotherapy because it can be directed to one part of the body. Still, it may cause severe scarring that can interfere with future organ function." To reduce collateral damage to healthy tissue hit by the radiation, without losing the impact on the cancer cells:

- *Ashwaganda* herb and vitamin E are significant protectors of healthy cells, yet increase tumor cell killing by radiation. Other radioprotectant agents to consider are quercitin, vitamin A, beta carotene, vitamin B3 - niacin, vitamin C, selenium, glutathione, squalene, alkylglycerols, genestein, curcumin, green tea, melatonin, zinc aspartate, taurine and ginseng.
- To reduce the chronic fibrosis and late effects I prescribe vitamin E 1000 I.U., vitamin C 1000 mg, milk thistle, and omega 3 fats from harp seal oil to be taken life-long.
- The traditional Vietnamese herb for detoxification *Vigna radiata* contains the flavenoid *vitexin* which has been shown to protect from radiation induction of weight loss, and damage to peripheral blood cells. Note that this herb treats the condition called "deficiency heat" seen by doctors of traditional Chinese medicine (TCM) in irradiated patients.

RADIOTHERAPY ENHANCERS

To increase cancer cell killing by radiation, and enhance chances of a cure:

- Maitake PSK, ashwaganda, melatonin, and vitamins A, C & E.
- PKC inhibitors regulate p-glycoprotein which acts as a pump to export drugs out of cells as well as acting as radiosensitizers, increasing cell sensitivity to radiation : hypericin, quercitin, apigenin, genestein are natural medicines which do this.
- COX-2 inhibitors selectively radiosensitize tumors, eg curcumin.
- Nicotinamide is a form of vitamin B3 which increases blood flow to tumors to overcome hypoxic cancer cell resistance to radiation. The effect is very specific to tumor vasculature. I worked for years in research on this problem of hypoxia or low oxygen levels in tumors. When a cancer grows faster than its blood supply some areas get starved and die off by necrosis. These low oxygen areas are places cancer cells can hide out and survive radiation therapy. After many millions of dollars spent on research, no drug is safer and more effective as a radiosensitizer than nicotinamide.

PRIMARY RADIATION SIDE-EFFECTS & MANAGEMENT TECHNIQUES

BURNS – *Aloe vera*, vitamin E, *Rosa mosqueta* oil, or Red Capital ointment may be used on burned skin. To prevent burning use aloe cream on the skin during the radiation treatment and after the treatment reapply it. Rosa cream prevents and treats burn scars. Use Ferlow Brothers aloe or rosa creams, in a base of organic grapeseed oil.

DISCOLORATION - vitamins A and D3 topically and orally

NERVE DAMAGE - acupuncture, vitamins B12, B6 and alpha lipoic acid; consider homeopathic *Hypericum* as well as the botanical form.

DESQUAMATION - vitamin E oil may be sprayed on sloughing skin

FAT NECROSIS - alkylglycerols from shark liver oil 600 to 1,200 mg daily

ANEMIA - bone marrow damage takes 1 to 3 weeks to manifest, but then may progress to complete anaplastic anemia - which is failure to produce any of the blood cell types. If the marrow stops making red blood cells the patient becomes anemic. Lack of red cells means not enough hemoglobin to carry oxygen out to the tissues and carbon dioxide back to the lungs to be breathed out as waste. Anemia makes a person tired and listless. Use iron with caution as it is very oxidizing, making ROS which damage DNA. It is best to check iron status by measuring serum ferritin before giving iron. Usually we need to support the bone marrow nutrition with sesame oil - 1 tsp.; shark liver oil alkylglycerols; *Marrow Plus* from Health Concerns - 3 to 4 capsules three times a day; *Shih Chuan Da Bu Wan* or Shiquan - 8 pellets three times
a day; Korean ginseng – 500 to 1000mg. twice daily.

LEUKOPENIA - failure to produce white blood cells means a loss of immune cells, so the person's resistance to infection can plummet. We naturopathic doctors have long had great success rebuilding immune health with thymus and spleen glandular extracts. I especially like to use Dolisos brand homeopathic *Thymuline*. My American colleagues like *Polyerga* spleen peptides. Botanicals to consider are *Astragalus* and *Phytolacca* - 30 drops of tincture twice daily, and *Eleutherococcus senticosus* - 300 mg. once a day. We may give dilute intravenous hydrochloric acid. We always recommend regular exercise. Avoid crowds, avoid people with infectious illness, and wash your hands often, especially after using the toilet and before eating. Report to your physician any sign of infection such as fever over 38° C, chills, cough, sore throat, painful urination, inflammation (redness, swelling) or pain in any area of the body.

THROMBOCYTOPENIA - failure to make platelets can make it impossible to form a clot, with a risk of severe hemorrhage. *Yunnan Pai Yao* (pseudoginseng) - 1 to 2 capsules three to four times daily is a reliable and fast therapy which I have seen outperform synthetic drugs. The pineal gland hormone melatonin may help regulate the production of platelets. Avoid aspirin (ASA) and Advil (ibuprofen), *Ginko biloba*, and other blood thinners. Report to your physician any bleeding signs such as bruising, red spots on skin, bloody urine or black, tarry stool.

FATIGUE - exercise, and start prior to therapy! The Chinese ginseng root *Panax ginseng* is a wonderful tonic, especially the liquid vials with royal jelly from China – take one to two vials daily, or in capsules take Pine tree brand royal jelly with ginseng. Naturopathic physicians may give intavenous "Myer's cocktail" of vitamins and minerals to revitalize and boost the immune system. I like to use Pascoe brand *Calycast* injectable ginseng extract with vitamin B12. Sometimes one must just conserve energy and ask for assistance on treatment days. Prepare food ahead of time and bank some down time - then use it to rest, contemplate, and visualize positive results from the therapy.

COLLATERAL ORGAN DAMAGE - beam collimation & masking take time, so make sure you ask the radiation oncologist to do this - remember the squeaky wheel gets the grease. You do not have to be embarrassed to remind your care givers to slow down and focus on your safety. You will be less hassle to them if you prevent problems before they occur. Use radioprotectants such as green tea, vitamin A, melatonin, glutathione and ashwagandha. Organs need supplemental Co-Q10 to repair - and it really makes a huge difference in healing.

PNEUMONITIS - lung irradiation can result in inflammation leading to fibrosis (scarring) which becomes acute 1 to 6 months after treatment, causing cough with blood in the sputum, shortness of breath, chest pain, and even death. Give patients at risk high doses of vitamin E, vitamin C, N-acetyl cysteine and milk thistle. Medical treatment includes prednisone, azathioprine or cyclosporine A.

NAUSEA - ginger root is very good - 2 capsules of root powder, grated ginger tea, or even as ginger ale. SeaBand is an acupressure band with a button that presses on PC-6. Even more potent is acupuncture needling at the points ST-36, PC-6, HT-1, CV-12. Homeopathic medications *Arsenicum*, *Nux vomica*, *Tabacum* or *Cuprum* have often worked very well. Eat often in small amounts, drink plenty of fluids. Medical marijuana (cannabis tetrahydrocannabinols) does work well for some, if they can tolerate the other effects. Allopathic drugs: Zofran, Compazine.

VOMITING - treat dehydration aggressively - drink electrolyte replacement, make a cup of miso soup, consider acupuncture. Replace salt and soda as well as water, or the water will not stay in the blood; the basic electrolyte replacement formula is ½ tsp salt, ¾ tsp baking soda, up to 8 tsp sugar and a cup of juice per litre water.

DIARRHEA - BRAT diet (banana, rice, apple, toast). L-glutamine acts as a food for the lining of the gut. Replace probiotic gut bacteria. Bentonite clay can absorb toxins. 'Prosperity treatment' is a special acupuncture technique using 4 needles around the belly button, and it can treat either diarrhea or constipation, with good results in about 5 minutes. *Po Chai* pills are the greatest Chinese herb formula for toxic diarrhea. Other possible supplements include CLA, vitamin A, fiber, glutathione, and omega 3 oils - cod liver oil deserves special mention.

CONSTIPATION - Hoxsey herbal tincture, high fiber, cod liver oil, Prosperity acupuncture treatment, good hydration, and an old naturopathic remedy called #42's which are capsules of cape aloe root and wormwood. #42's are remarkable for relieving even the most stubborn constipation from codeine and morphine painkillers.

MUCOSITIS - sores and ulcers in the mouth or anywhere in the gastrointestinal tract are improved with the amino acid L-glutamine dosed up to 6 gm/day, liquid folic acid, glycyrrhiza, chamomile tea or tincture, chlorophyll, ulmus, vitamin E gel, and *Radiacare* oral rinse. Use a very soft toothbrush, or a finger or gauze pad, and consider baking soda rather than toothpaste. Avoid crunchy, spicy and acid foods. A simple oral rinse of ½ teaspoon each of baking soda and salt in a glass of warm water may be used several times a day. The mouth will be soothed by cold or frozen yoghurt and soft, bland food.

ANOREXIA - loss of appetite is helped by ginger, bitters, peppermint, thiamine, melatonin, *Marinol*. Make small meals, and control odors.
Be aware that bromelain can powerfully inhibit appetite.

CACHEXIA - 80% of cancer cases are malnourished, and 40% die of malnutrition. Weight loss must be monitored and managed aggressively. Loss of over 20% lean body mass is critically dangerous; increase carbohydrates & protein intake. Use EPA oils e.g. cod liver oil 1 Tblsp. up to twice daily, melatonin, L-glutamine, bitter melon *Momordica charantia*. The prescription drug hydrazine sulphate can be helpful, as it inhibits gluconeogenesis.

CHEMOTHERAPY

For a few generations now, whenever a really poisonous substance was found in nature or made in a drug laboratory, it was immediately sent to the cancer research establishments to be evaluated as a cancer drug. The orthodox or allopathic medical treatment of cancer has emphasized *cytotoxic* or cell-killing medications. Chemo drugs kill rapidly dividing cells, targeting their DNA. Most of the cytotoxic effect results from apoptosis triggered by sublethal DNA damage. This is good. However, they also tend to go beyond this level of damage into *necrosis,* the rapid death of cells, which is a messy, inefficient and risky process, producing inflammation which is itself a promoter of tumor growth.

"Chemo" side-effects limit dosage, limit efficacy, and even kill patients. Any step we can add which reduces these risks increases the potential for the chemo to achieve its intended result. I consider it a major success to help a patient live through chemo with a reasonable reserve of health. As Dr. Robert Atkins, M.D. has said in *Atkin's Health Revolution,* "The damage done to the body by an unsuccessful course of chemotherapy is often so great that the patient's immune system never recovers sufficiently to stand a fighting chance." Naturopathic physicians confirm this observation, that if chemo is given and fails, the hope for a response to biological treatments is also likely lost. We just too often have nothing left to work with in these damaged bodies.

Chemo drugs obey first-order kinetics - a constant percentage of cells are killed by a given exposure, i.e. if a drug kills 99.999% and the tumor burden is a billion cells, there will be 10,000 surviving cells, causing an apparent clinical remission but guaranteeing a reoccurrence in time. It is nearly impossible for chemo to kill every last cancer cell.

Chemo is more effective with leukemias and lymphomas than with solid tumors, possibly due to drug delivery issues. In the disseminated cancers chemo is so successful you would be daft to not try it. Other than these blood-borne cancers, and testicular cancer, which are only 3% of all cancers, chemotherapy is not well proven to good scientific standards to have a positive influence on survival or quality of life. This is well known to oncology doctors, 75% of whom say they would not participate in a chemotherapy trial if they had cancer, due to its "ineffectiveness and its unacceptable toxicity". Yet in North America 75% of cancer patients are prescribed chemo by these same doctors. In Canada, the same 75% majority of oncologists surveyed said they "would not undergo chemotherapy or recommend it to a loved one" for a majority of cancers!

This sort of nonsense has cost the medical profession a lot of credibility with patients. Ultimately, we must have *integrity* – to be one and the same to all persons, all the time - to fulfill our professional duty to each patient. There are hard choices, to be made between the doctor and patient, in an atmosphere of trust. The question I ask myself with patients is would I take the treatment myself, or give it to my children or my dear wife. I wonder if most oncologists could answer this question truthfully with their patients. In some states such as California and New York, it is illegal for a physician to treat cancer by any method other than chemotherapy drugs, surgery and radiation! God save us when the Queen and her courts get involved in our health care!

Fractionated chemo - using small doses more often over a longer time - tends to give better outcomes, as do multi-drug protocols. Other techniques to improve the risk to benefit ratio include intra-arterial infusions, chemo resistance screening tests, monoclonal antibody chemo targeting, and chromotherapy light-activation. A naturopathic doctor I know had the same osteosarcoma that cost Terry Fox his leg, but he was in the USA. He had the chemo delivered in extremely high doses into his leg, but while the blood to his leg was isolated from the rest of the body and run through a heart-lung bypass to keep it oxygenated. He is alive and walking on both his legs a decade later.

Cells lacking a functioning p53 gene cannot undergo apoptosis after chemo. This applies to 50 % of cancers, especially late stage. Old tumors mutate and develop resistance to these drugs. Support apoptosis with vitamin E, berberine, quercitin, green tea, curcumin and antioxidants.

Chemo is commonly toxic to other rapidly growing normal cells - bone marrow , epithelium, GI mucous membranes, hair follicles - thus causing anemia through loss of replacement red blood cells, loss of platelets needed for clotting, loss of white blood cells of the immune system, baldness, nausea, diarrhea, vomiting, GI and mouth ulcerations, and so on. Heart damage, nerve damage, kidney damage, infections due to immune suppression, tinnitus, and pneumonitis, are also frequent problems. Many patients get 'chemo brain' syndrome - confusion and mental deterioration. Chronic late effects include persistent fatigue, persistent bone marrow suppression, infertility, and increased risk of other cancers such as leukemia and lymphoma.

Multi-drug resistance develops in cancer cells treated with chemotherapy, and so tumors which develop after the primary therapy are very hard to treat. Dangerous advanced tumors are made less resistant to chemo by bioflavenoids like quercitin.

TREATING COMMON CHEMO TOXICITIES

Expectation plays a central role in the occurrence of side-effects. If the patient believes they can stay well, visualizes success, and positively affirms and embraces the therapy, they will likely do better than if they are fearful. However, it is not a trivial concern that chemo can cause great harm, even death. Anxiety is therefore normal, but high levels of depression, as measured by the Hospital Anxiety and Depression Scale (HADS) questionnaire, can predict pathological responses to chemotherapy. Such patients may display high emotional restraint and not appear severely depressed. This is a good reason to integrate mind-body medicine with orthodox protocols! After chemo most patients will benefit from both detoxification for health restoration, and tonification of their fundamental vitality.

ANEMIA - bone marrow damage takes 1 to 3 weeks to manifest, but then may progress to complete anaplastic anemia - which is failure to produce any of the blood cell types. If the marrow stops making red blood cells the patient becomes anemic. Lack of red cells means not enough hemoglobin to carry oxygen out to the tissues and carbon dioxide back to the lungs to be breathed out as waste. Anemia makes a person tired and listless. Use iron with caution as it is very oxidizing, making ROS which damage DNA. It is safer to check iron status by measuring serum ferritin before giving iron. Usually we need to support the bone marrow nutrition with sesame oil 1 tsp., shark liver oil alkylglycerols, *Marrow Plus* from Health Concerns 3 - 4 capsules three times a day, *Shih Chuan Da Bu Wan* or Shiquan 8 pellets three times a day, *Panax ginseng* 500 to 1000 mg. twice daily. *AHCC* (active hexose correlated compound) is a proprietary Japanese low molecular weight compound from fermented shiitake and other medicinal mushrooms grown in rice bran, which has been found to prevent many chemo side-effects and increase the effectiveness of methotrexate, 5-fluorouracil and cyclophosphamide at doses of 3 grams daily.

LEUKOPENIA - failure to produce white blood cells means a loss of immune cells, so the person's resistance to infection can plummet. Naturopathic doctors have long had great success rebuilding immune health with thymus and spleen glandular extracts. I really like to use Dolisos homeopathic thymus *Thymuline* or *Polyerga* spleen peptides. Botanicals to consider are *Astragalus* or *Phytolacca* 30 drops of tincture twice daily, and *Eleutherococcus senticosus* 300 mg daily. We may give dilute intravenous hydrochloric acid. Avoid crowds, avoid people with infectious illness, and wash your hands often, especially after using the toilet and before eating. Exercise. Report to your physician any sign of infection such as fever over 38ºC, chills, cough, sore throat, painful urination, or inflammation such as redness, swelling and pain anywhere.

THROMBOCYTOPENIA - failure to make platelets can make it impossible to form a clot, with a risk of severe hemorrhage. *Yunnan Pai Yao* (pseudoginseng) 1 - 2 capsules three to four times daily is a reliable and fast therapy which I have seen outperform drugs. The pineal gland hormone *melatonin* may help regulate the production of platelets. Avoid aspirin (ASA) and Advil (ibuprofen), *Ginko biloba*, and other blood thinners. Report to your physician any bleeding signs such as bruising, red spots on skin, bloody urine or black, tarry stools.

NAUSEA - ginger is very good, as 2 capsules of root powder, as tea, even as ginger ale. SeaBand is an acupressure band with a button that presses on PC-6. Even more potent is acupuncture needling at the points ST-36, PC-6, HT-1, CV-12. Homeopathic *Arsenicum*, *Nux vomica*, *Tabacum* or *Cuprum* have often worked very well. Allopathic drugs: Zofran, Compazine Eat often in small amounts, drink plenty of fluids. Medical marijuana (cannabis tetrahydrocannabinols or THC) does work well for some, if they can tolerate the other effects.

VOMITING - treat dehydration aggressively - drink electrolyte replacement, make a cup of miso soup. Consider acupuncture such as PC-6. Replace salt and soda as well as water.

DIARRHEA - BRAT diet (banana, rice, apple, toast). L-glutamine gives energy to heal to the lining of the gut. Replace probiotic gut bacteria. Bentonite clay can absorb toxins. Prosperity treatment is a special acupuncture technique using 4 needles around the belly button, and it can treat both diarrhea or constipation, with good results in about 5 minutes. *Po Chai* pills are the greatest Chinese herb for toxic diarrhea. Consider also vitamin A, CLA, fiber, glutathione, omega 3 oils; cod liver oil deserves special mention.

CONSTIPATION - Hoxsey tincture, high fiber, cod liver oil, Prosperity treatment, good hydration, and an old naturopathic remedy called #42's which are capsules of cape aloe root and wormwood. #42's are remarkable for relieving even the stubborn constipation from codeine and morphine painkillers.

ANOREXIA - loss of appetite is helped by ginger, bitters, peppermint, thiamine, melatonin, marinol. Make small meals, and control odors. Be aware that bromelain can powerfully inhibit appetite.

DEHYDRATION - treat aggressively with electrolyte drinks and miso broth; ½ tsp salt, ¾ tsp baking soda, up to 8 tsp sugar, and up to a cup of fruit juice to 1 liter water for a dehydrated patient. Intravenous normal saline, 0.9% salt, with 5% glucose.

CACHEXIA - 80% of cancer cases are malnourished, and 40% die of malnutrition. Weight loss is a cardinal sign of cancer, and must be monitored and managed aggressively. Loss of over 20% lean body mass is critically dangerous; increase carbohydrates & protein intake. Use EPA oils e.g. cod liver oil 1 Tblsp. up to twice daily, melatonin, L-glutamine, bitter melon *Momordica charantia*. The drug hydrazine sulphate can be helpful to block gluconeogenesis.

MUCOSITIS / STOMATITIS - sores in the mouth and bleeding gums hurt, reduce eating and can get infected. Use L-glutamine at to 6 gm/day or 2 gm/m², liquid folic acid/folate, *Glycyrrhiza* as DGL licorice extract, chamomile tea or tincture, *Calendula* succus (marigold juice), chlorophyll, *Ulmus* (slippery elm bark), vitamin E gel, and *Radiacare* oral rinse. Use a very soft toothbrush, or a finger or guaze pad, and consider baking soda rather than toothpaste. Avoid crunchy, spicy and acid foods.
A simple oral rinse of ½ teaspoon baking soda and salt in a glass of warm water may be used several times a day. The mouth will be soothed by cold or frozen yoghurt and soft, bland food.

FATIGUE - exercise - and start prior to therapy! The Chinese ginseng root *Panax ginseng* is a wonderful tonic. I like the liquid vials with royal jelly and reishi from China – take one to two vials daily, Naturopathic physicians may give intavenous 'Myer's cocktail' of vitamins and minerals to boost the immune system and revitalize. Sometimes one must just conserve energy and ask for assistance on chemo days. Prepare food ahead of time and bank some down time - then use it to rest, contemplate, and visualize positive results from the therapy.

NEUROPATHY - L-glutamine 6 to 10 grams a day, vitamin B6 500 mg twice a day, vitamin B12, B-complex, calcium, antioxidants, milk thistle, and alpha lipoic acid at least 200 mg. daily. Burning mouth syndrome is a toxic neuropathy shown to respond very well to alpha-lipoic acid.

KIDNEY DAMAGE - repair any organ damage with Co-enzyme Q10, in doses of 100 to 300 mg daily. Renal tubule damage is helped by quercitin at about 1,500 mg daily. Support it with mixed anti-oxidants.

HAND-FOOT SYNDROME - palmar-plantar erythrodysthesia (PPED) begins as a tingling, numbness or redness of the skin on pressure areas such as hands, feet, elbows or knees. It can progress to severe reddening and peeling of the skin at the extremities, which can impair function and lead to serious infections. Use aloe topically and take vitamin B6.

SELECTIVE TOXICITIES OF SPECIFIC CHEMOTHERAPY AGENTS

VINCA ALKALOIDS - Vincristine and Vinblastin from periwinkle bind tubulin, destroy mititic spindles, causes constipation, paralytic ileus (small bowel paralysis), alopecia (baldness), stomatitis, dermatitis and neurotoxicity (foot drop, paraesthesias, loss of tendon reflexes)

- Effectiveness is increased by vitamin A, vitamin C and vitamin E.
- Prevent or treat neurotoxicity with milk thistle, vitamin B6, vitamin B12 and alpha lipoic acid. Give stool softeners or laxatives.

ETOPOSIDE - *Podophyllum* alkaloid toxins are enhanced with melatonin, vitamin A, and beta-carotene.

CYCLOPHOSPHAMIDE (CP) - Cytoxan is a mustard alkylating agent which cross-links DNA, potentially causing nausea, alopecia, hemorrhagic cystitis, myelosuppression (bone marrow damage).

- Increase effectiveness with vitamin A, beta carotene, vitamin C, vitamin E, coenzyme Q10, folic acid, quercitin and aloe vera juice.
- Reduce toxicity with ashwagandha, melatonin, N-acetyl cysteine, glutathione, Polygera spleen extract and lots of water.

BISULPHAN - synergistic with quercitin against human leukemia

CISPLATIN & CARBOPLATIN - platinum complexes which cross-link DNA, and deamidates the Bcl-xL gene, which inactivates a switch that could trigger apoptosis. Platinum compounds can cause severe neurotoxicity, severe nephrotoxicity (kidney damage), nausea, vomiting, ototoxicity (hearing loss) and myelosuppression. Monitor electrolytes for low sodium, calcium, potassium and magnesium

- Improve effectiveness with gluathione 800-2,000 mg, quercitin 1,500 mg, coenzyme Q10, gingko biloba 120 -240 mg, milk thistle 600 - 900 mg, selenium 400 - 800 mcg, PSK 3,000 mg, lentinan, vit. A, C and D.
- Reduce toxicity with gingko biloba (renal and nerve protectant), milk thistle (liver protectant), quercitin, selenium, glutathione, melatonin, all-trans retinoic acid (ATRA), alpha lipoic acid, Polygera, and vitamins C and E. Low vitamin E status correlates with severe peripheral sensory neuropathy from cisplatin. Carboplatin is less renal toxic but more myelosuppressive than cisplatin; produces electrolyte imbalances, nausea and vomiting, abnormal liver function, neuropathy, myalgia (muscle pain) and is mutagenic. Consider extra glutamine and Polygera with carboplatin.
- Do <u>not</u> mix platinum drugs with N-acetyl cysteine, zinc or high dose vitamin B6.

5-FLUORO-URACIL (5-FU) - a pyramididine anti-metabolite which inhibits DNA synthesis which causes anorexia, nausea, stomatitis, diarrhea, alopecia, renal failure, leukopenia, rashes, pigmentation changes - darkening and sunburning easily. This is an "anti-vitamin" agent.

- Improve effectiveness with quercitin, melatonin, aloe vera, shitake lentinan and vitamins A, vitamin C, vitamin E.
- Reduce toxicity with glutamine, glutathione, chamomile mouthwash, coenzyme Q10, and vitamin B6.
- Caution: do not mix with high doses of carotenoids, including beta carotene, lutein, and lycopene.

DOXORUBICIN - Adriamycin is an anthracine antibiotic which intercalates DNA (binds inside the spiral strands), inhibiting DNA and RNA synthesis and can cause chromosome breaks. It is highly toxic to the muscle of the heart over total doses of 500 mg/m2. Doxorubicin is a pro-oxidant, causes myelosuppression with leukopenia and post-treatment acute myelocytic leukemia (AML), alopecia, nausea, vomiting, and extravasation (leaking of fluid out of the blood vessels).

- Use caution mixing with N-acetyl cysteine or glutathione antioxidants as they can interfere with the antitumor activity.
- Improve effectiveness with vitamin A, beta carotene, vitamin C, vitamin E, DHA, milk thistle, green tea, curcumin, quercitin and genestien.
- Reduce toxicity with garlic, selenium, coenzyme Q10, melatonin, curcumin, catechin and vitamins A, beta carotene, B2, B6, C & E.

Anti-oxidants in virgin olive oil also seem to help.
Vitamin B6 particularly reduces hand-foot syndrome (PPED).

METHOTREXATE (MTX) - is an antimetabolite or anti-vitamin agent which inhibits dihydrofolate reductase, blocking reduction of the B-vitamin folic acid, necessary for DNA nucleic acid and protein synthesis. It is sometimes given in a fatal dose followed by 'leucovorin rescue' which is calcium folinic acid. MTX is nephrotoxic and hepatotoxic (damages the kidneys and the liver). It causes nausea, vomiting, diarrhea, mucositis (mouth sores), dermatitis (inflamed skin), blurred vision, dizziness, and leukopenia (drop in immune white blood cells).

- Improve effectiveness and reduce toxicity with vitamin A, vitamin E, selenium and L-glutamine. Glutamine increases uptake of MTX into tumors.
- Do not combine with glutathione, tangeretin, or high doses of folic acid or vit. C.

EPIRUBICIN - is less toxic to humans given melatonin supplementation.

BLEOMYCIN - is less toxic and more effective in patients given supplemental vit. A.

TAXOL - mitotic inhibitors in yew tree bark taxanes can produce anaphylactic shock reactions, commonly treated with Benadryl and/or Decadron - an antihistamine and a steroid drug. Sensory neuropathy, myalgia, arthralgia, mucositis, nausea, vomiting, leukopenia and cardiac toxicity can also occur. Proactively control hypersensitivity.
- L-glutamine at 10 gm up to three times daily reduces risks of neuropathy and myalgia.
- Vitamin C - 4 to 6 grams daily improves efficacy.
- Do not mix with berberine, quercitin or St. John's wort as they may reduce efficacy.

TAMOXIFEN - is a non-steroidal anti-estrogen which binds to cytoplasmic estrogen receptors, and has other complex effects on hormones. It causes blood clots, hot flashes, retinal damage, rashes, leukorrhea, depression, liver damage and can increase tumor pain. In the presence of bony metastases it can precipitate hypercalcemia (excess blood calcium). It increases risk of uterine cancer to 1 t0 3 per 1000 cases.
- Melatonin is highly synergistic and reduces risks by reducing cytokines and reinforcing hormone blockade.
- GLA oil at 2.8 grams daily improves effectiveness
- vitamins A, C & E improve effectiveness.
- Do not combine with soy foods or soy isoflavones, flavenoids such as tangeritin or grapefruit, black cohosh root *Cimicifuga racemosa*, St. John's wort *Hypericum perfoliatum*, or red clover blossoms *Trifolium repens*, including Hoxsey herbal tonic.
- Smoking should be stopped and alcohol minimized.

THALIDOMIDE - a potent inhibitor of angiogenesis, it may also be useful for cachexia. May cause neuropathy, treatable with vitamin B6 100 mg or more and alpha lipoic acid 100 mg or more, both three times daily.

GEMCITABINE - quercitin reduces tumor cell resistance.

TOPOTECAN - quercitin reduces tumor cell resistance.

CARMUSTINE (BCNU) - beta-glucans from maitake mushroom increase efficacy against prostate cancer by inhibiting a glutathione dependent detoxifying enzyme glyoalase I (Gly-1).

PREMETREXED – less toxic if homocysteine levels are reduced, so give B12 , folate.

Several foods and natural herbs in common use can interact poorly with chemotherapy drugs, by inducing liver enzymes which clear the drugs. This can increase toxicity or result in therapeutic failure. There is no confirmed data, but some things to consider avoiding during chemo: St. John's Wort, grapefruit, garlic, rosemary, alcohol, tobacco, and yohimbe.

In chemotherapy, no matter what drug, always consider supporting with:

1. *Shih Chuan Da Bu Wan* 12 pellets twice daily to restore bone marrow

2. Green cabbage and mung bean sprouts juiced, for appetite and to protect the lining of the gut. *Fare You* "vitamin U" cabbage extract pills can be used too.

3. Royal jelly and *ginseng* with *ganoderma* for fatigue & immunity.

4. *Ashwagandha* 1 to 2 capsules 2 to 3 times daily

5. Vitamin A 10,000 I.U. daily

6. *Polyerga* - spleen peptides 300 to 500 mg daily

7. DHA (docosahexanoic acid) fatty acids from fish and fish oils or from seal blubber oil.

DETOXIFICATION STRATEGIES

Detoxification is important after chemotherapy, in cancer prevention and health maintainence.

The liver is the primary organ of detoxification. Any synthetic, toxic or otherwise biologically useless molecule must be removed by turning it into a form which can be breathed out via the lungs, sent out in the bile and out the colon as feces, sweat out through the skin, or eliminated by the kidneys in the urine. In Phase 1 the liver oxidizes the compounds to make a reactive site. The mixed function oxidase enzymes are supremely adaptable. However, they can make the compounds they are working on even more toxic than before. In Phase 2 of liver detox, the reactive sites are bound or conjugated to various small molecules, most of which are amino acids or sulphur compounds. This generally renders them inert and ready to dispose of.

The basic naturopathic approach to detoxification emphasizes:

- lots of purified water, preferably micro-cluster magnetized water
- fresh organic fruits and vegetables, whole, juiced, steamed or lightly cooked
- fibre supplements such as ground flaxseed and psyllium husks
- bitter herbs for the liver such as dandelion root, burdock root, globe artichoke, Russian black radish, Oregon grape root, and milk thistle. Other good herbs include parsley, nettle, celery seed - as in Seroyal brand *Herbotox* tablets.
- omega 3 fats with DHA as in fish and seal oils.
- adequate protein - use fish, and if needed add hydrolyzed whey.
- supplemental antioxidants - vitamin C, alpha lipoic acid, selenium, N-acetyl cysteine, glutathione, vitamin E and grapeseed extract OPC.
- body cleansing such as enemas, colonic irrigation, infrared sauna, castor oil packs, peat or mud baths, and constitutional hydrotherapy.

The castor oil pack - This home treatment relieves pain and congestion in the abdomen, is a strong stimulator of lymphatic drainage, and detoxifies the liver. Wool flannel is soaked with castor bean oil - *Oleum ricini* - and applied over the tummy, covered with plastic, and a heating pad or hot water bottle applied over it for about one hour. Repeat as needed. Clean up with 3 tablespoons of baking soda in a liter of warm water.

Constitutional hydrotherapy - The ultimate naturopathic hydrotherapy, perfected by Dr. Otis Carroll, ND This treatment uses electrical stimulation along with wraps of cold and hot packs, and takes about an hour or more. It is repeated until there is a cleansing reaction. It is proven to detoxify and to stimulate immune function. This is true naturopathy, working to assist the body to heal in the most gentle way.

THE SEVEN DAY BROWN RICE DIET

- Eat when hungry, all you want of organic brown rice, fresh vegetable or fruit juices, steamed vegetables, ocean fish, skinless free-range chicken, soy (tofu, miso, tempeh), lentils, humus, rice cakes, sesame seeds, onions and garlic.

- A vegetable broth made from root vegetables and greens is an alternative to juices.

- The very best vegetables are beets, garlic, onions, cabbage, brussell sprouts, spinach, parsley and squash.

- For seasoning use ginger, garlic, parsley, rosemary, cilantro, cayenne pepper or non-salt herb mixes.

- Avoid oranges, catfish, shellfish, red meat, eggs, dairy, fatty foods, wheat.

ROUTINE DETOX

It was customary in earlier generations to do a regular Spring clean-out by purging with sulphur and molasses, castor oil, or other laxatives, along with a few days on a vegetable or liquid diet.

There are even more toxins in our food and water now than ever before, and thousands of new artificial chemicals enter our environment every year. We have electromagnetic pollution, a faster pace of life, economic pressures, and so many other stresses on our system.

I believe in doing something daily to try to keep these negative influences moving on out of my body, and suggest you do the same. This includes fibre supplements such as psyllium husks and fresh ground flaxseed with probiotic bacteria, liver herbs such as milk thistle or *Herbotox* formula, purified water - spring, glacier, distilled or reverse osmosis, adequate clean protein - vegetarian, organic meat or whey isolates.

Detoxification also applies to the mental and emotional aspects of our lives, and our relationships with others. Exercise, playing gentle music, and mental hygiene such as meditation also help. The best thing a person can do for themselves is to find a way to give selflessly to others. Love is a magical healing force.

Chapter Four -   DIET & SUPPLEMENTS IN CANCER

"The scientific and medical literature and theorists fail to vividly portray issues which are patently obvious to clinicians, especially those who work with nutrition."
            Dr. Mark Gignac, N.D., Cancer Treatment Centers of America

Many nutrients are associated with lowered risk of certain cancers, and are therefore preventative. Most are antioxidants and flavenoids, some are minerals, vitamins, proteins and oils. They abound in the traditional foods of our ancestors that can be hunted, milked, fished, picked or gathered.

Lowered risk from all cancers, and longer survival with cancers, is associated with low caloric intake. Over-eating is a major risk that is all too commonly taken in our modern society with its energy rich agricultural foods. Overfueling causes insulin resistance, hyperinsulinism, hormonal shifts, blood fat imbalances, and metabolic aging. Periodic fasting extends the human lifespan.

Good nutrition naturally supports healing as well. Dietary interventions with cancer patients appear to remove obstacles to cure.

There are about 200 documented cases of spontaneous remissions from advanced cancer each year in the U.S.A. These often correlate with dietary factors, including a switch to vegetarian diet and use of supplements. The Grape Cure, Gerson Diet Therapy, the Macrobiotic diet, Dr. Kelley's Nutritional Metabolic Therapy, Dr. Brusch's Diet, the Hallelujah Acres - God's Way Diet and Moerman Diet all have their supporters, and may be useful adjuncts to more definitive therapies.

The clinical bottom line is that diet alone may not cure cancer, but bad nutritional management will contribute to reduced repair and healing, weight-loss, cachexia, fatigue and complications. Malnutrition and ination (not eating) are the direct cause of death in 22% of all cancer patients.

The absolute taboos in the diet of cancer patients are high sugar foods and red meat raised by contemporary agribusiness methods. We forbid tobacco products. I strongly urge reduction of chemical intake in all forms, by washing food better, choosing organic food, raising your own food, and by cleaning up chemicals in the home and workplace. Beyond this point we need to get personal, and tailor the diet to the individual constitution, tastes, culture, condition and disease.

The modern agricultural-based diet is significantly different from the diet of our hunter-gatherer ancestors. Our ancestors had very low rates of cancer. The protective elements they had which we now tend to lack in our diets are largely due the reduction in consumption of coarse vegetation, especially the herbaceous or aerial parts of plants. These lost protectants include calcium, potassium, fibre, omega 3 fatty acids, polyunsaturated fats, trace minerals, antioxidants, flavenoids, isoflavones and polyphenols.

For example, covalent DNA binding is inhibited by phenethyl isothiocyanate in broccoli and cabbage, ellagic acid in fruits, nuts, berries, seeds and vegetables, and by polyphenolic acid flavenoids in fruits and vegetables. Tumor promoters are inhibited by retinol and carotenoids in orange, yellow and green fruits and vegetables, vitamin E in nuts and wheat germ, organosulphur compounds in garlic and onions, curcumin in tumeric (curry) and by the vanillyl alkaloid capsaicin in chili peppers.

Estrogen, progesterone and thyroid hormones are biotransformed into benign forms by indole-3-carbinol in cabbage, brussel sprouts, broccoli, cauliflower and spinach, and by selenium in garlic and seafoods.

Absorption of carcinogens is reduced by fiber in fruits, vegetables, grains and nuts, and by riboflavin and chlorophyll in fruits and vegetables.

The modern diet is an experiment in nutrition which is not going well for us. The hybridized plants that are now staples in our diet have been genetically manipulated to be big and sweet and juicy, release more sugar faster because they have simpler starches and less fiber.

Foods may be heavily contaminated with chemical carcinogens and xenobiotics. Our estrogen and insulin growth factors are going wild!

Grain silage and "by-product" (filth) fed animal foods are also higher in compounds associated with higher cancer risk, such as xenobiotics, saturated fat, herbicides and pesticides.

Until wholesome nutrition is at the core of cancer therapy and prevention, the disease will remain unbeatable.

GERSON THERAPY

Dr. Max Gerson, M.D. developed a diet of primarily raw foods, with emphasis on fresh juices of vegetables, fruits. He gave his patients Lugol's iodine solution, pancreatin enzymes for digestion, thyroid extract, mineral and vitamin supplements. He prescribed raw calf liver either orally as a juice or by injection! He was often able to arrest or even regress metastases, although he less often saw clearance of the primary tumors. He published the book *The Gerson Therapy, Results of Fifty Cases* describing cured cases, but was labelled a quack. His clinic was forced out of the U.S.A. and now operates in Tijuana, Mexico, under the direction of his daughter Charlotte. Dr. Steve Austin, N.D. was my professor of nutrition and of oncology at National College of Naturopathic Medicine in the early 1980's. He has conducted a preliminary independent survey of the results of the Gerson approach. The diet takes great effort to make everything fresh throughout the day, and actual compliance falls off quickly once the patient returns home. However, even with excellent compliance, results are startlingly poor. Dr. Austin says about Gerson patients "All they do is the therapy, they don't have a life. It's not worth it".

I must acknowledge potassium iodide is worthwhile, that raw foods provide needed potassium and enzymes, and that raw liver is an excellent tonic for the fatigued cancer patient. However, the Gerson diet is just too cumbersome and too radical to be of practical importance to the average patient. Ditto macrobiotic diets.

ISSEL'S THERAPY

Josef Issels described cancer as a series of multiple and chronic challenges and insults. Issels combined a variety of techniques to adapt to the individual patient and their current status. For over 50 years he used Coley's toxins, a non-specific mixed bacterial vaccine. The patients for whom it provoked periodic fevers saw regression and resolution of tumors. He also used a specific autologous vaccine made from mycoplasma and related organisms found in the patient's own blood. He emphasized correction of the pro-malignant milieu, tumor debulking, and host support. He often removed tonsils and teeth as sources of focal infections and toxicity.

SUGAR, BLOOD GLUCOSE, INSULIN & CANCER RISK

- High dietary sugar intake is associated with many cancers, including breast, colorectal, biliary and melanoma. The worst sugar is sucrose from sugar cane. Sucrose, fructose and many other food sugars are mostly converted into glucose, the major sugar found in the blood stream, and the primary energy fuel for most cells in the body.

- Insulin is a protein made in the pancreas and put into the blood to move fats, sugars and proteins into cells. It must attach to the receptors on the cell membrane in order to pump nutrients into the cell. Its attachment is assisted by glucose tolerance factor (GTF), which is composed of chromium, zinc, and some B-vitamins. Insulin increases fat storage and therefore promotes excess body fat. Insulin also activates the liver enzyme HMGCoA reductase to overproduce cholesterol from carbohydrates. Exercise and stress reduction lower insulin levels.

- Insulin resistance is a complex metabolic problem where the insulin cannot get nutrients into the cells. Insulin resistance is linked to increased incidence of cancer of the colon, breast, pancreas, esophagus, uterine endometrium, and prostate. A marker for insulin resistance is the apple-shape body type with prominent abdominal obesity. Insulin resistance can also lead to "Syndrome X" with high blood pressure, cholesterol disorders, cardiovascular disease - atherosclerotic plaque, stroke and heart attacks, and other major health risks such as osteoporosis, osteoarthritis, and premature aging.

- Cancer patients increase glucose production in the liver by 25 to 40%, similar to non-insulin dependent adult onset diabetics (NIDDM), also known as type 2 diabetes. Unlike diabetics, cancer patients will continue to increase sugar production even while undergoing starvation, accelerating loss of body mass.

- Cancer cells metabolize glucose sugar at a rate 4 to 5 times that of normal cells.

- When there is not enough oxygen to burn sugars in the usual way, cancer cells switch to fermentation. Fermentation is not very efficient, making about 20 times less energy from the sugar than if it were burned in the usual way by oxidation, and leaving more harmful residues in the process. Lactic acid from fermentation is highly toxic and a tumor growth promoter.

- Malignant tumors have 1.9 to 3.0 times the insulin and related compounds seen in normal tissue.

- Insulin is a general growth promoter. Hyperinsulinism and insulin resistance are highly pro-inflammatory, increasing IL-6, C-reactive protein, and NF kappa-B. Hyperinsulinism is seen in about 45% of early cancers, but rises to about 75% of advanced cancer cases.

- C-peptide is a marker for pancreatic insulin secretion, accurately reflects the mean level of circulating insulin, and associates with cancer risk.

- Chronic hyperinsulinism and insulin resistance increases delta-9-desaturase activity, which alters the ratio of stearic to oleic fatty acids, which may contribute to post-menopausal breast cancer.

- Post-prandial hyperinsulinemia - high blood insulin after eating - produces a signifigant surge in the doubling rate of hepatocellular carcinoma cells, which last for several hours after a meal that spikes up the blood sugar. Insulin excess in the bloodstream is not consistently correlated to the glycemic index of the foods due to great individual variability in digestive function and absorption faculty.

- Insulin-like growth factor one (IGF-1) or somatomedin C is a mitogenic peptide which promotes cell proliferation, anabolism, clonal expansion and inhibits apoptosis. IGF-1 is involved in the decision by the cell to progress from G-0 to G-1 phase of the cell cycle. Elevated levels are associated with a several fold increase in risk of ovarian, prostate, colorectal and lung cancer. Insulin inhibits IGF binding proteins (IGFBP 1 & 2) and this increases IGF bioavailability. Free IGF-1 may stimulate estrogen receptors. Insulin and IGF may be directly mitogenic, interact with ras protein mutations, stimulate farensyl transferase, modulate apoptosis, and stimulate angiogenesis by increasing production of vascular endothelial growth factor. IGF-1 is excessive in milk from cows given recombinant bovine growth hormone (rBGH). IGF signalling is suppressed by vitamin D analogues - another good reason to take your cod liver oil and get some sunshine. IGF-1 is also inhibited by green tea EGCG.

- A relatively new alternative therapy is the use of high doses of insulin to induce a hypoglycemic state in the cancer cells. This is risky, but does potentiate other therapies.

WEIGHT LOSS & METABOLIC CACHEXIA

Cachexia is the wasting away of the body triggered by metabolic changes of cancer. It is far more than just loss of appetite (anorexia) and digestive power. It is a critical shift into a chemical imbalance where the body consumes itself to feed the tumor with nitrogen and other elements. It is a cause of great distress, weakness, and robs the person of dignity. It is often manageable, which can prevent premature death and suffering.

- Involuntary loss of 5% of lean body mass in the past 3 months or a 10% weight change in the past 6 months is a high risk negative prognostic indicator.

- Tumor products such as lipid-mobilizing factor (LMF) directly stimulate lipolysis (fat burning) in a cAMP dependent system, and proteolysis factor initiates catabolism of skeletal muscle. Both respond well to eicosapentanoic acid (EPA) supplements such as fish oil or seal oil. Fish or seal oil EPA is the most effective supplement to manage weight loss, at 2 grams EPA daily. I like to use harp seal oil, 2 capsules daily, or cod liver oil, up to 1 tablespoon daily. Salmon oil can be used, but it goes rancid too fast for me to be comfortable with it.

- Cachexia is also triggered by host immune factors such as the cytokines IL-1, IL-6, INF-gamma and TNF-alpha.

- Tumor necrosis factor alpha (TNFa) produced by macrophages, lymphocytes and NK cells, is also called *cachectin* because it causes anorexia and weight loss, via the hypothalamic satiety center in the brain and by inhibition of gastric emptying. It increases glucose uptake, insulin resistance, protein catabolism in skeletal muscle, depletes fat stores, and is associated with fatigue. TNF also induces reactive oxygen species, which are involved in tissue wasting. TNF can be inhibited by green tea epigallocatechins (EGCG), eicosapentanoic fatty acid (EPA), melatonin, vitamin E succinate (VES), and the botanicals *Uncaria tomentosa* (cat's claw) and *Silybum marianum* (milk thistle).

- Progesterone has a proven track record of benefiting appetite, body weight and subjective well-being. It is presumed to down-regulate the synthesis and release of cytokines. It can stimulate prostate and breast cancers to grow.

- Ling Zhi Feng Wang Jiang is a pleasant and effective nutritive general tonic for the qi and blood, strengthens and invigorates the fatigued cachexic patient. The active ingredients are ginseng, royal jelly and ganoderma mushroom. It can restore appetite, nutrient and medication absorption, and body weight. Take one 10 ml. vial every morning, and another later in the day if needed. If they are very Yang deficient combine this with Chinese ginseng *Panax ginseng*, or Siberian ginseng *Eleutherococcus senticosus* 500 mg to 3 times daily.

- Thalidomide has shown some potential benefits on appetite, nausea and well-being. Other drugs being studied are Ibuprofen at 50 mg twice daily to reduce C-reactive protein; pentifylline I.V. to reduce TNFa; and COX-2 inhibitors celecoxib or rofecoxib to modulate prostaglandins involved in cachexia as well as in the development of cancer. There are many natural COX-2 inhibitors. See page 146.

- Corticosteroids are used to inhibit prostaglandins and to suppress TNF production. The results on appetite, food intake and quality of life are short-lived, and there are significant risks of adverse effects. Steroids are best reserved for end-stage palliation.

- The drug hydrazine sulphate was developed by Dr. Joseph Gold to stop the cachexic process. It was the first non-toxic chemotherapy developed, only causing some nausea and limb weakness in some cases. It is very inexpensive. It inhibits gluconeogenesis, slows or stops tumor growth, and produces significant improvement in subjective symptoms in at least half of terminal cases - in other words patients just feel better, have less pain, more energy, and increased appetite. Despite strong science from America and Russia, the cancer institutions such as the National Cancer Institute and and the American Cancer Society have systematically blocked research efforts and have marginalized this drug. This sordid behaviour is a triumph of politics over truth, to maintain the power and income of those who have entrenched interests in surgery radiation and toxic chemotherapy.

PROTEIN & CANCER

Be vigilant, protein intake is a huge modifier of outcomes. Tumors become nitrogen sinks by catabolizing skeletal muscle, recruiting amino acids for gluconeogenesis via the lactic acid Cori cycle. Protein will then be drawn from the patent's flesh.

L-glutamine - is a principle fuel of cancer cells, generating 30 ATP energy molecules per glutamine. It is a critical stimulant of protein and nucleic acid (DNA and RNA) synthesis. L-glutamine protects the body from ammonia build-up, absorbing this toxic by-product of proteins, acting as a "nitrogen shuttle" to divert ammonia into amino acids, amino sugars, urea, nucleotides and the super-antioxidant glutathione. It protects the gut lining from radiation and chemotherapy, suppresses prostaglandin PGE2 synthesis, stimulates NK natural killer cells. It reduces gut absorption and permeability changes and diarrhea caused by 5-fluorouracil. It protects from taxane neuropathy. L-glutamine is used medically in healing from surgery, injury, sepsis (widespread infection), and starvation. It is not commonly found in intravenous feeding (total parenteral nutrition - TPN) solutions as it rapidly hydrolyzes so supplement with up to 30 grams daily by mouth or add to a parenteral bag for cachexia. Even 2 grams can make some difference. L-glutamine is very useful to reduce cravings for alcohol. It is critical to immune competence against infection, fuelling neutrophils, monocytes lymphocytes, improving the Th1/Th2 ratio.

Serum albumen - under 3.5 is high risk, and survival falls 33% for every point decrease. Serum albumen falls with metastases, liver disease, expanded serum volume, and renal dysfunctions, so it does not just reflect loss of lean body mass. Serum half-life of albumen is 3 weeks.

Alpha-lactalbumin - in human breast milk induces apoptosis in malignant trophoblastic cells in the infant digestive tract.

Whey protein - lactalbumine in cow's milk is an excellent source of supplemental protein for cancer patients. Take 1 ounce or 30 grams of powder in liquid drink twice a day. Whey strips glutathione out of cancer cells, but raises it in normal cells!

SeaGest - is a peptide concentrate from fresh lean white fish of the North Pacific, at 12 to 20 capsules daily for wound healing, to arrest cachexia, and for general vitality. The fish is bioconverted to peptides and amino acids by bacterial fermentation. Assimilation is nearly 100%.

Haelen - is a nitrogen enriched fermented soy protein drink developed in Chinese hospitals to supercharge their cancer patients with protein.

MINERALS

SELENIUM - is strongly associated with cancer prevention at 200 mcg daily, and is a useful antioxidant therapy at 400 to 800 mcg.
Selenium may be an inhibitor of angiogenesis.

CALCIUM - at 1,200 mg daily reduces proliferation, assists redifferentiation, binds unconjugated bile acids.

MAGNESIUM - correlates with protection from prostate cancer, and inhibits the secretion of insulin.

ZINC - is antiangiogenic by reducing copper absorption. Zinc induces metallothionein, an endogenous tumor promoter. Enhances apoptosis and DNA repair mechanisms. Zinc deficiency has been linked to squamous cancers. Too much zinc increases cancer risk.

IRON - supplements are pro-oxidant, tend to stimulate tumors and can aggravate bacterial infections. Do not give unless the serum ferritin is confirmed to be below normal.

POTASSIUM - salts are perhaps the most critical mineral in controlling normal cell function, and it is absolutely certain that our ancestors ate a lot more potassium than does modern man. The agricultural diet has inflicted a huge reversal of the ratio of sodium to potassium seen in hunter-gatherer diets.

Potassium is found in all vegetables, and it is a good idea to drink the water in which vegetables are cooked. Excellent food sources are potatoes and bananas.

From Dr. F.W. Forbes Ross in early twentieth century London, to the Americans Professor Andrew C. Ivy, Dr. Max Gerson, and Harry Hoxsey in our time, the use of potassium iodide, potassium citrate, and potassium phosphate has been associated with cancer cures.

POTASSIUM IODIDE - is routinely used at 5 grains weekly, or about 50 mg daily. Certainly it is generally safe in these dosages, as it has long been used at twice this dose as an expectorant for coughs. Sometimes a patient will experience *Iodism* - pimples on the face, forehead or shoulders, watering eyes, and a runny nose. Rarely, allergic reactions can occur, with vomiting, cramps, fever, palpitation, and emaciation. Potassium iodide will pass in breastmilk and will cause nursing babies to lose weight.

IODINE - as found in potassium iodide, is a tonic to the thyroid gland. Low thyroid is associated with poor immune function and healing. Hypothyroid is also linked to constipation, which is very detrimental to a cancer patient. I have seen patients pulled back from the brink of death by getting their bowels moving, and the relief of pain that accompanies this is also remarkable. The thyroid interacts in complex ways with sex hormone balance. For example, we will use iodine supplements to reliably get rid of fibrocystic breast lumps. The recommended dose of elemental iodine is 350 to 375 micrograms daily. See the comments on *iodism* given above in the discussion of potassium iodide.

Dr. Max Gerson felt that iodine counteracts the neoplastic effects of hormones! Iodine is used to make thyroid hormone, which sets the body thermostat, and how fast all the metabolic systems will run. Adequate thyroid function is critical to detoxifying the body of toxins produced by cancer cells, by the often toxic therapies for cancer, and especially to clear off the wastes and cell fragments as cancer cells die from a good therapy. Even natural therapies can result in a huge burden on the reticulo-endothelial system and liver detox systems, so it is critical to support the body in throwing off the diseased tissue. Potassium iodide was found in the Hoxsey formula at 3% W/V. Gerson used Lugol's iodine solution or dessicated thyroid extracts.

DIETARY FIBER

- Associated with lower risk of colorectal cancer.
- Pre-agricultural "hunter-gatherer" diets were very much higher in fiber than modern diets.
- Carrier of phytoestrogens which are anti-estrogenic.
- Diminish re-uptake of sex hormones, binds hormones and carries them out in the feces.
- Lignans and isoflavenoids in food fibre stimulate production of sex hormone binding globulins (SHBG) which bind free estrogen.
- IP-6 or phytic acid up-regulates p21 and p53 genes while down-regulating mutant p53. Blocks tumor initiation and progression. At 5 to 8 grams daily it may inhibit breast and colon tumor growth. Phytic acid strongly chelates dietary minerals and medications, so take fiber away from all medicines.
- Used by gut bacteria to make butyrates and other beneficial short chain fats.
- Take a daily fiber supplement such as psyllium husks and ground flaxseed.

DIETARY FATS

Low fat diet <u>before</u> diagnosis is associated with 70% lower risk of mortality in breast cancer cases; changing to low fat diet after diagnosis has no measurable survival benefit. While it may be too little too late, a reasonably low fat diet with a balance of fats is healthful and may reduce risk of heart disease, stroke, diabetes, and most other diseases.

Tumors increase fatty acid oxidation and lipolysis to provide the gluconeogenesis substrates glycerol and free fatty acids. This allows them to make energy without sugars.

GOOD FATS

- Extra virgin grade (cold-pressed) olive oil has the omega 9 monounsaturated oleic fatty acid, squalene and phenolic antioxidants known to protect against cancer of the breast, colon or skin. Oleic acid inhibits conversion of AA to PGE2. In prostate cancer this conversion is ten times that in benign prostatic hypertrophy (BPH or enlarged prostate gland).

- CLA from meat and milk of grass-fed animals. Conjugated linoleic acid (CLA) inhibits tumor initiation and reduces metastases at 1% of dietary calories. CLA is cytotoxic and cytostatic, modulates cellular responses to tumor necrosis factor alpha, enhances cell-to-cell communication, reduces hyperinsulinemia, benefits cachexia, and increases IL-2 production. Loading dose is 100,000 to 3,000,000 units. There is a small risk of dry skin, headaches and changes in liver enzymes.

- monosaturates and gamma linolenic acid (GLA) from nuts and seeds. GLA is associated with induction of cAMP, which redifferentiates cancer cells, and restores contact inhibition. Evening primrose oil or borage oil are good sources.

- omega 3 fat as found in soy, canola, walnut, almonds, flaxseed, fish, and fish liver oils - especially eicosapentanoic acid (EPA) and dihexanoic acid (DHA). EPA reduces PGE2 production, alters other cytokines and prostaglandins, reduces cachexia, inhibits platelet aggregation, inhibits metastasis, promotes apoptosis, modify cell-cell signalling, and improves immune helper-suppressor cell ratio.

SHARK LIVER OIL

Shark liver oil contains alkylglycerols which are powerful stimulants to humoral and cellular immunity, including a marked effect on NK cell activity. It helps recovery from bone marrow suppression after chemotherapy. Animal studies show a great synergy with probiotics. Use 6 of 200 mg capsules for up to 30 days maximum, as it may over-stimulate platelet production.

BUTYRATES

Butyrates are short chain fatty acids found in butter and made from fibre in the gut by friendly bacteria. Butyrates stabilize the DNA and genetic code, and induce re-differentiation in colorectal and other cancers. Butyrate is a very important nutritional supplement for all cancer patients. Its taste and odor is similar to rancid butter, which some find objectionable. These salts of butyric acid can be made with sodium e.g. *TriButyrate* sodium 4-phenylbutyrate, potassium or other minerals. Butyrates are formed naturally in the gut by friendly bacteria (probiotics) digesting fibre, such as the fibre in psyllium seed husks.

CALCIUM-D-GLUCARATE

A salt of glucaric acid, calcium-D-glucarate (CDG) naturally occurs in citrus fruits such as oranges and in vegetables such as the *Cruciferae* (cabbage family) and potatoes. It also is naturally produced by friendly gut bacteria in the colon or large intestine, where it inhibits beta-glucuronidase activity. CDG increases net elimination of fat soluble carcinogens, toxins, steroid hormones. Glucarate increases glucoronidation in Phase II liver detoxification pathways, lowering lipids, regulating estrogen metabolism, decreasing estradiol levels, preventing hormone dependent cancers such as breast, prostate and colon. Human dose range is 1.5 to 3 grams daily, e.g. 3 capsules 1 to 2 times daily of Tyler brand, a professional product line.

BAD FATS

Arachidonic acid (AA), trans-fatty acids, excess omega 6 fatty acids (corn, soybean and safflower oils), excess linolenic acid (LA), saturates. The omega 6 fats are too high in the modern Western diet, such as from corn oil in margarine and shortening, and in meat fed on corn silage. Trans fatty acids (TFA) in hydrogenated oils and polyunsaturated fatty acids (PUFAs) are pro-oxidants and promote mutation. Too much TFA's are common in any oil that has been over-heated, especially in frying foods or grilling. PUFA's go rancid fast and do not stand up to cooking either.

VITAMIN D3

The active form of vitamin D. Vitamin D is partly activated in the kidney and becomes fully active as a vitamin and hormone from sunshine on the skin.

- promotes normal cell differentiation, acts directly on DNA
- inhibits angiogenesis
- suppresses IGF-1 signalling
- promotes apoptosis
- helps bone metabolism, calcium absorption
- used topically, it can heal many skin disorders, even reversing early pre-cancerous lesions. For this purpose mix in vitamins A and C too.

Supplement at 800 to 1,600 I.U.

High dose vitamin D therapy can provoke *hypercalcemia*, and increase risk of kidney stones. Monitor closely and ensure a good fluid intake!

VITAMIN A

Vitamin A palmitate and other retinoic acids are regulators of epithelial cell growth, and important immune modulators. Vitamin A penetrates into the very nucleus of the cell to receptors sites which regulate the normal growth and diferentiation. This is where the action is in a cancer cell. It is safe in doses up to 50,000 I.U. daily.

- promotes apoptosis
- promotes cell differentiation
- highly protective against viral infection
- decreases serum insulin-like growth factor1 (IGF-!)
- inhibits 5-alpha reductase, reducing testosterone levels
- upregulates transforming growth factor beta
- improves tumor response to radiation and chemotherapy
- protects the gut from chemotherapy
- prolongs survival in advanced cancers
- retinoic acid reduces viral DNA inside cells

COD LIVER OIL

Pure cod liver oil is a tremendous food for cancer patients. It has been used medically for over 200 years. It supports the immune system and healing.   It is rich in vitamin A, vitamin D, squalene, EPA and DHA, all of which are antineoplastic. EPA is very effective in preventing loss of skeletal muscle in cancer patients.   Vitamins A & D are also immune stimulators. Take 1 to 2 tablespoons daily.

REVICI'S LIPIDS

Emanuel Revici, MD was an innovative and revolutionary thinker who developed non-toxic therapies for cancer and other diseases. Revici began researching the role of fats in cellular metabolism in the mid-1920's, and continued this work in Manhattan at the Institute of Applied Biology from 1947 to his death in 1998 at the age 101 years. He made house calls at the age of 100!

He tested urine pH to individualize "biologically guided chemotherapy" based on the normal daytime acidification from catabolic processes and the nightly alkalinity from anabolic processes. He described the catabolic phase as increasing entropy by electrostatic charges and fatty acid predominance. He described the anabolic phase as quantum forces which oppose degeneration and increase order. Anabolism provides "negentropy" or negative entropy, opposition to the tendency of all things to become unorganized and dispersed. Anabolism is directed by sterols such as estrogen, progesterone and adrenal hormones. Recall that body builders use anabolic steroids to bulk up. The opposite of anabolism is catabolism, the actions in the body which break down materials or cells. He used "guided lipid" therapy to balance any extreme of either phase, consisting of fatty acids, sterols, animal tissue extracts and minerals incorporated into lipids. His opus was the 1961 text *Research in Pathophysiology as Basis for Guided Chemotherapy with Special Application to Cancer.*

This work is being carried on by Dr. Lynn August, MD who continues research on creating food grade fats as medicines. Fundamental to her work is the thesis that the fats at the cell membrane are the final defense of the immune system, and that cellular fats regulate the cell's behaviour and health. Dr. August runs a consultation service called Health Equations which interprets standard medical blood tests to yield 'biological indices' of the relative dominance of catabolism (breaking down), anabolism (building up), and other aspects of metabolism. Even if all the lab values for a patient are in the "normal" range, some indicies may be outside a range that is consistent with stability and balance. As a general rule of thumb a lab value that is within one third of the range from the middle of the normal values to the limits of normal is within the ability of the homeostatic control mechanisms to keep things stable. However, in the outer two thirds of the normal range there is increasing instability. When several biochemical pathways become unstable, risk of disease can become significant. Thus the analysis can show degenerative tendencies so preventative corrective action can be taken before gross illness occurs. The emphasis is on correcting the diet with whole foods, and if necessary, nutritional supplements.

Revici's belief in the health value to the immune system of natural cholesterol in foods such as meat, eggs and butter is echoed in the work of Diana Schwarzbein, MD in her excellent dietary book *The Schwarzbein Principle*. Many chronic diseases such as diabetes, autoimmune diseases, cardiovascular disease, arthritis and cancer were not common in cultures which ate a lot of these now politically incorrect foods. Recall the "French Paradox" which is a low rate of heart disease in French people eating a lot of cheese, butter and meat cholesterol. As in all things, it is the balance and quality of the foods in the diet which is the real issue.

I certainly believe in the "Paleolithic Diet" principles, that we should eat the way our ancestors did, whole foods that could be taken from Nature by picking, gathering, digging, hunting, fishing, milking. This Stone Age style of eating is proven to result in less cancer, heart disease, stroke, and auto-immune diseases than the modern agricultural foods diet.

We need fear what the farmer does to the animal, not meat itself. Wild game is a health food. Grass fed domesticated animals are nearly as good.

A chicken allowed to live the life allotted to a chicken by its Creator is a wonderful food, on which our races have thrived, until man was put in charge of feeding them.

It is time to admit that veterinary and nutritional science has led us down the garden path and is spoiling our animal foods as certainly as chemicalization is despoiling the environment at large. Until they can show modern agri-business is decreasing and reversing the horrendous rates of cancer we are facing, most people will reasonably remain suspicious of the latest creations.

We are eating our way into our hospitals, and into our graves. This human tragedy is millenia old now, but it can be halted. Food should be life. Natural living foods shall be your medicine.

ANTIOXIDANTS

Always use mixtures! Single anti-oxidants are like drugs - unbalanced and unnatural. Take them the way they are found in Nature, working together as a team to detoxify, fight infection, and to rejuvenate. They work together in a beautiful synergy.

Oxygen began to be available in the environment when bacteria developed blue-green pigments for photosynthesis. Later these tricks passed to algae as the little miracle of chlorophyll, which takes light and stores it into chemical energy. Now all plants use the technology, store the sun as food for all other living creatures, and release oxygen. Oxygen makes up 21% of the air we breathe.

Oxygen reacts with almost every other element. It "oxidizes" by moving electrons, making high energy compounds. Oxygen chemistry makes possible the higher life forms which are very active. However, it not only reacts, it burns. To keep it in check, plants make a lot of antioxidants, which squelch its harsher characteristics. When we have a good *redox* balance between the forces of oxidation and reduction, we enjoy the harmonious state of good health. Plant foods give this balance in our human bodies.

Antioxidants induce selective apoptosis of cancer cells, leaving normal cells unharmed, induce differentiation in cancer cells, making them behave more normally, and reduce cancer cell proliferation - so tumors grow more slowly.

Oncologists have been arguing that antioxidants are risky with chemotherapy since reactive oxygen species formed in chemotherapy are downstream mediators which may be needed to trigger apoptosis.   In other words the doctors think taking vitamins and anti-oxidants might stop their drugs from working to kill cancer.   However, there is no science to prove this hypothesis.   This does not stop scientists from promulgating the fear of mixing safe vitamins with dangerous drugs. They err on the side of leaving patients under-nourished and subject to the full brunt of the drugs anti-nutrient effects. Why? The political and economic system sees nothing much to gain from researching something which anyone can make and sell. If no big drug company wants to invest big money, no real work gets done. Scientists sell their services for research grants. No grants, no answers to simple questions, therefore no inclusion in evidence-based medical practice. However, it is not actually the case that most of orthodox medicine is proven to a high standard to be safe or effective, nor is it true that naturopathic medicine is not supported by a wealth of good scientific evidence. We do need and welcome more research, however.

Do we even need high end research to tell us foods that prevent cancer and support health and healing processes are good for cancer care?

The fact that antioxidants actually help patients feel better, and in fact they help them to survive, is easily brushed aside as anecdotal and observational evidence. It is still evidence, and until better evidence is put forward, is clinically relevant.

Reducing oxidative stress during chemotherapy shifts cell killing from necrosis towards apoptosis. Caspase activation and apoptosis follow cytochrome C release from mitochondria, which is an early event in cancer cells undergoing chemotherapy, therefore cancer cells may be committed to apoptosis well before ROS (reactive oxygen species or free radicals of oxygen) are generated. ROS also inhibit caspases, enzymes which disassemble the cell once pro-apoptotic signals are given. Anti-oxidants would de-inhibit the caspases, so would tend to drive apoptotic cancer cell killing.

Anti-oxidants may actually help promote apoptosis, may protect normal cells from the drugs, and may help coordinate the entire sequence. Naturopathic physicians use antioxidants discreetly with drugs, as there are a few poor interactions. However, good research evidence of good interactions support our clinical observations. I hope in time enough science is done to validate this approach to the satisfaction of all.

There is a paradoxical pro-oxidant effect which some so-called anti-oxidants exert under some circumstances. The answer to this problem is to have lots of various types of anti-oxidants to create balance. These wonderful vitamins seem capable of doing whatever is best for the cell and the body, as long as they are in the balance found in whole foods.

High fat diets often have a lot poly-unsaturated fatty acids (PUFA's) which are already rancid from reacting with air or can oxidize within the body. PUFA oxidation forms strongly electrophilic aldehydes which bind to cysteine-rich extracellular domains of death ligand receptors. Antioxidants prevent PUFA oxidation, so the death receptors can stay open for business - and kill cancer cells.

Apoptosis after radiation and chemotherapy agents depend on death ligand receptors. Antioxidants can help many chemotherapy agents,
X-ray and hyperthermia treatments ligate or tie into these receptors -
in other words, helps them kill cancer cells.

Properly selected and combined antioxidants reduce the toxicity of these treatments to normal cells, protecting your health.

VITAMIN C

- Vitamin C or ascorbic acid increases peroxide poisoning of cancer cells. Tumors produce less than normal of the catalase enzyme which removes naturally occurring peroxides, allowing a deadly build up of hydrogen peroxide (H_2O_2).

- Vitamin C is also anti-apoptotic, inhibiting caspase-9 activity and suppressing induction of apoptosis by TNFa and angiotensin II.

- Vitamin C improves mitogen responses and increases production of IL-2.

- Vitamin C is very effective in reducing chemical toxicity to DNA and to the liver.

- In moderate doses it alters hyaluronidase activity, slowing the spread of cancer.

- Doses of 500 to 1,000 mg are as effective as 5,000 mg doses to increase NK cell activity, reduce apoptosis and increase mitogenesis of immune cells, restoring functionality to the immune system. Large oral doses can cause gas and crampy intestinal pains.

- Used palliatively, in large IV doses, it will extend life in terminal patients. At 400 mg/dl it is cytotoxic. Linus Pauling promoted use of really high intravenous vitamin C, up to 50 grams a day. It did arrest some cancers, but there were also some deaths from internal bleeding. This is likely from the sudden lysis or dissolving of tumors - perhaps it worked too well. Because of this danger it is the policy of most naturopathic physicians to only go this high in terminal cases, where the benefits may outweigh the risks. It is clear from the Mayo Clinic studies that patients who have had extensive chemotherapy are not as responsive to high dose vitamin C as those who have not had their immune system ravaged by these drugs.

- Vitamin C can also act as a *pro-oxidant*, and so is the most problematic antioxidant if high doses are combined with many of the chemotherapy drugs.

- Taper off high dose regimes slowly to avoid rebound scurvy.

GLUTATHIONE

GSH is the most powerful antioxidant substance, critical to good immune function, particularly against viral infection.

- induces normal p53 activity by redox modulation, which induces apoptosis in tumors.
- is a protectant in radiation and chemotherapy.
- detoxifier from alcohol, drugs, tobacco, pesticides, herbicides, xenobiotics, petroleum hydrocarbons, smog, pollution, heavy metals, many carcinogens and tumor promoters.
- glutathione is protected and regenerated by anthocyans as found in grapeseed extract, and interacts in an antioxidant network with selenium, vitamin C, vitamin E and alpha lipoic acid.
- is made from the amino acid cysteine, found in protein foods.
  Milk whey protein has the glutathione precursor cystine. Recall that alpha-lactalbumin in fresh human milk induces apoptosis in malignant trophoblastic cells.
- glutathione is given in doses of up to 1,600 mg daily. Oral doses may be partly digested by protein dissolving digestive enzymes, but some may be absorbed intact. Use sublingual lozenges.
- some naturopathic physicians provide intravenous administration of orthomolecular doses of pure glutathione in a normal saline drip. Recent evidence casts doubt on the effectiveness of this approach. Oral precursors are safe - NAC, whey, HMS 90.

N-ACETYL-CYSTEINE

NAC is a supplement which can be converted in the body into the ultimate antioxidant cancer fighter glutathione (GSH).

- a significant lung protectant, and markedly thins excess mucus. It has long been used in treating emphysema, asthma, bronchitis, tuberculosis. Use it anytime the lung is affected by cancer or by cancer treatment, such as radiation therapy.
- elevates p53 activity and apoptosis in cancer cells
- supports liver detoxification in Phase 2 conjugation reactions.
- suppresses NFkB activity, as does GSH and vitamin C.
- inhibits viral transcription and boosts cellular immunity
- directly inhibits TNFa.
- chelates out toxic heavy metals and copper.

VITAMIN E

Vitamin E is a family of compounds called tocopherols and tocotrienes, which are fat-soluble anti-oxidants. The most common natural form of vitamin E is d-alpha-tocopherol. Vitamin E compounds protect fats in cell membranes from oxidizing. When vitamin E levels are too low, the cell membranes get stiff and cannot pass nutrition in and wastes out.

- Especially as vitamin E succinate or VES, vitamin E promotes apoptosis, stimulates cell differentiation, inhibits angiogenesis, inhibits TNF.
- Vitamin E is protective against breast, colon and prostate cancer.
- Vitamin E increases the cytotoxic activity of 5-fluorouracil, doxorubicin and cisplatin by inducing p53. It reduces mucositis.
- Vitamin E is highly protective of lungs, brain and other high oxygen tissues.
- Vitamin E is very protective against radiation damage.

CAROTENOIDS

Beta carotene (provitamin A), lycopene, lutein, and other carotenoids in the diet are strongly associated with reduced risk of various cancers. There may be a therapeutic role in breast, prostate and cervical cancers. Lycopene reduces IGF-1 stimulation of cancer cell growth in hormone dependent tumors, and is best derived from cooked tomatoes. Lutein is found in spinach, broccoli, oranges, carrots, lettuce, tomatoes, celery and green vegetables.

GRAPESEED EXTRACT

Grapeseed ortho-proanthocyanidins - see botanical section.

....

Some cancer alternative pioneers thought some foods contained oxygen inhibitors, and thus reduced the ability to oxidize toxins: tomatoes, alcohol, coffee, lentils, beans, and meats. Certainly alcohol and coffee and other stimulants impair glucose tolerance and insulin sensitivity. Hoxsey and Koch warned against eating tomatoes, but we now know they are rich in lycopene and are associated with reduced rates of prostate cancer. Legumes were not a staple in pre-agricultural diets; their risk remains to be explored.

QUERCITIN

Quercitin is a natural polyphenolic bioflavenoid found in many foods and herbs, such as white oak bark, apples and onions. The average diet provides about 25 mg daily. It is the primary dietary bioflavenoid. Quercitin is 3,3',4',5,7-pentahydroxyflavone, a sugarless (aglycone) form of rutin, and it can easily oxidize to a quinoid form which is a redox agent. While it is very mutagenic, it is not thought to be carcinogenic, Bioflavenoids like quercitin do inhibit thyroid peroxidase, which adds the iodine to thyroid hormone, and will aggravate hypothyroidism in patients with inadequate iodine consumption. For this reason we may combine it with potassium iodide supplementation.

- an aromatase inhibitor, it reduces estrogen hormone formation in adipose tissue (fat cells). The aromatase gene CYP19 expression is promoted by prostaglandins sensitive to COX -2 inhibitors.

- binds type II estrogen receptors in breast, colon, ovary, melanoma, leukemia and meningeal cancer cells, inhibiting growth. ER-2 receptors have only a weak affinity for estrogen, and probably inhibit growth when stimulated by flavonoids. ER-2 expression is independent of ER-1 status, and the effective growth inhibition in breast cancer is equal to Tamoxifen.

- down-regulates expression of mutant p53 protein, arresting human breast cancer cells in G2-M phase of the cell cycle and human leukemia cells T-cells and human stomach cancer cells in G1-S phase. DNA replication is thus markedly reduced.

- inhibits heat shock proteins, which disrupts formation of complexes of mutant p53 and HSP's which would allow tumor cells to bypass normal cell cycle checkpoints. No HSP's means no mutant p53 activity. If HSP's are left unchecked there is a risk of shorter disease-free survival and increased chemotherapy drug resistance in breast cancer.

- enhances NK cell activity and is immune stimulating

- induces apoptosis; blocks tumor export of lactate, resulting in a lethal drop in tumor pH, triggering pH-dependent apoptosis endonucleases.

- cytotoxic effect is dose-dependent.

- inhibits high aerobic glycolysis of tumor cells and thus inhibits ATP synthesis

- inhibits cyclooxygenase and lipoxygenase, especially the 5-lipoxygenase/ 5-HETE eicosanoid pathway.

- inhibits DNA polymerases B and I.

- inhibits p21-ras proto-oncogene, which is a mutation found in 50% of colorectal cancers. The p21-ras mutation impairs cellular GTP-ase, allowing continual activation of the signal for DNA replication in colon cancer and many other tumor types.

- inhibits replication of RNA and DNA viruses

  - blocks peroxide inhibition of cell-cell signalling

  - suppresses signal transduction pathways such as protein kinase C and casein kinase II, preventing these signals from the cell surface to the nucleus from over-riding normal growth controls.

  - inhibits multidrug resistance

  - interferes with ion pump systems

  - inhibits metastasis

  - increases effectiveness of radiation and chemotherapy, especially doxorubicin, ribavarin and tamoxifen

My learned colleagues at the Cancer Treatment Centers of America (CTCMA) prescribe a quercitin combination *BCQ* - bromelain, curcumin and quercitin - from Vital Nutrients at doses of 2 capsules three times daily.

CURCUMIN

Curcumin is derived from the yellow curry spice, the tumeric root - *Curcuma longa* or *yu jin*. Dietary intake is protective against various cancers.

- induces apoptosis in cancers eg liver, kidney, sarcoma & colon

- highly chemoprotective, blocks tumor induction by chemical carcinogens, inhibits cancer initiation, promotion and progression

- antioxidant against superoxide, hydroxyl radicals, peroxynitrite.

- inhibits inducible nitric oxide synthetase by reducing its mRNA transcription

- decreases eicosanoids such as 5-HETE and PGE2 to strongly reduce inflammation

- prevents activation of NF kappa B

- stimulates the reticulo-endothelial immune system, activates phagocytosis by immune cells

- inhibits spontaneous DNA damage from lipid peroxidation

- induces heat shock protein hsp70 to protect cells from stress

- significantly inhibits angiogenesis

- significantly inhibits number and volume of tumors

- reverses liver damage from fungal aflatoxins and mutagens in tobacco smokers

- Vital Nutrients brand *BCQ* - 2 capsules 3 times daily provides curcumin with bromelain and quercitin. Canadians use professional products such as (AOR) brand, 1 to 2 of 500 mg capsules 3 times daily. Some naturopathic physicians like a combination of curcumin with black seed - the cumin spice seed Nigella sativa. TCM doctors may use 'Canelim' tablets with curcumin, and other herbs. Curcumin combines well with genestein from soy, synergistic with EGCG from green tea.

MELATONIN

Melatonin is the natural indoleamine hormone produced in the pineal gland in the brain. The daily variation in light received by the eye tells the pineal gland to make bursts of melatonin. In more technical detail: the enzyme N-acetyltransferase emitted in a circadian cycle from the suprachiasmatic nucleus after photic stimulation through the retinohypothalamic tract converts serotonin into melatonin.

This internal body clock, designed to work under natural light, makes a daily hormone tide which creates a biological rhythm.

Pinealectomy (removal of the gland) enhances tumor growth and metastasis in experimental animals. Pineal extracts, even if melatonin-free, inhibit human cancer cells.

Working rotating night shifts or going to bed after 2 am increases risk of breast cancer, presumably due to suppression of melatonin production.

Long-term safety as a supplement is well established - for example melatonin has long been used in Europe in oral contraceptives.

For insomnia and jet-lag we use 1 to 3 mg at bedtime.

For cancer we use 10 to 20 mg at bedtime. The dose is reduced if the patient has nightmares or feels dopey in the morning. After about 3 years of use the dose should probably drop to about 5 mg at bedtime.

Melatonin is very helpful in most cancers, not just hormone dependent types.

IMPORTANT NOTE: <u>Never</u> take melatonin at any other time than at bedtime - what we call "the hour of sleep" - in the late evening. This is an example of chronobiology, the timing of administration of medicines to match natural daily biological cycles.

IMPORTANT NOTE: There is a small theoretical risk of interaction if combined with SSRI antidepressant drugs such as Paxil - it could provoke serotonin syndrome, with a sudden rise in blood pressure.

IMPORTANT NOTE: Avoid melatonin for patients with disseminated cancers such as leukemia, lymphoma and multiple myeloma.

Melatonin is a balancer and stabilizer in all stages of solid tumors:

- improves survival time as a sole agent in terminal cancer.
- doubles survival time and response rate to conventional therapy in all hormone sensitive cancers.
- antioxidant, protecting DNA and cellular membranes from oxidation.
- inhibits cancer initiation, anti-carcinogen.
- modulates hormones - estrogen, testosterone, prolactin and may make tumors more hormone dependent, which is more amenable to treatment
- blocks mitogenic effects of hormones and growth factors
- increases effectiveness of radiotherapy, reduces myelodysplasia
- decreases cell proliferation directly
- increases gap junctional intercellular communication
- controls fatty acid uptake, transport and metabolism.
- increases apoptosis
- modifies cytokines, increasing host immune defenses via thymus and T-helper cell derived opiod peptides.
- decreases circulating cytokine interleukin 6 (IL-6) significantly
- down-regulates 5-lipoxygenase gene expression
- increases p53 expression
- reduces TNF secretion, reduces cachexia with metastatic solid tumors
- increases response and survival with chemotherapy - reduces myelosuppression (bone marrow damage) and thrombocytopenia (loss of platelets needed for blood clotting).
- synergistic with IL-2, increases effectiveness up to ten fold, allowing use of only 10% of the usual dose
- synergistic with Tamoxifen
- naturally increases with meditation (focused awareness exercises).

CO-ENZYME Q10

CoQ10 or ubiquinone is a fat soluble antioxidant critical to cell energy production.

- intestinal absorption is poor, and may limit effectiveness
- may improve survival in several types of cancer; early studies show dramatic regression rates in advanced breast cancer - in combination with selenium, B-complex, vitamins C & E, betacarotene, EFA's and magnesium – at doses from 90 to 390 mg daily.
- CoQ10 is absolutely a must for any organ failure, such as congestive heart failure or kidney failure as induced by chemotherapy drug poisoning.

ALPHA LIPOIC ACID

- water and fat soluble thiol antioxidant
- increases glutathione - GSH activity
- NFkB inhibitor at about 600 mg daily
- blocks heat shock proteins
- powerful therapy for all forms of neuropathy - from chemo or diabetes.
- Many naturopathic physicians use Poly-MVA, a trimeric palladium lipoic complex with vitamins thiamine and B12.

CATECHIN

- bioflavenoid, increases activity of antioxidant enzymes
- inhibits formation of adhesions after surgery
- inhibits mutagenesis and carcinogenesis
- induces apoptosis in a dose-dependent fashion
- inhibits tumor growth
- arrests malignant cells in G0-G1 phase of cell cycle
- enhances wild type p53 expression
- inhibits protein kinase C activation by tumor promoters

INDOLE-3-CARBINOL

- I3C naturally occurs in cruciferous *Brassica* vegetables, including broccoli, cabbage, cauliflower, brussel sprouts, kale and watercress. These foods are strongly associated with broad cancer protection.
- I3C is released by chewing, converts to diindolylmethane (DIM) in stomach acid; DIM is more stable than I3C and may be the better supplement.
- decreases 'bad' 16-OH and 4-OH estrogens by 50%
- increases 'good' 2-OH estrone and estradiol by 75%
- down-regulates estrogen receptor activity
- induces apoptosis, regulates apoptosis genes, arrests cells in G1

I rely on the professional Tyler brand *Indoleplex* DIM, 2 capsules at bedtime for women; 4 capsules at bedtime for men or Thorne Research Indole-3-carbinol, dosed at 200 to 400 mg daily. These reliably reduce PSA in prostate cancer, and are of great service in breast cancer. I-3-C and DIM are also useful for other hormone overload problems such as acne, premenstrual tension, menstrual disorders and menopause.

GARLIC

Allium sativa or garlic is a great health food. It is the best immune building food, and promotes longevity.

- immune tonic *par excellence*
- detoxifier
- anti-angiogenic because it boosts nitric oxide synthesase activity
- diallyl disulphide (DADS) from the breakdown of allicin alters cancer cell metabolism of proteins and polyamines, cell cycle and adhesion properties.
- chemoprotective, anti-proliferative anti-mitotic and tumor shrinking effects have been observed with garlic extracts.

When I was 24 years old, and in good shape, I was invited by an older local man to climb up a large hill to a ruin of an oracle temple in Greece. I could not keep up with him, which disturbed me because he appeared he could be 60 years old. After turning back several times to goad me on, he threw me a head of garlic and advised me to eat a few cloves. He said this is why he was so strong in his 80's! I will never forget how impressed I was with his vigor, and I have no doubt his advice to eat lots of garlic every day was very wise. Anyone beginning to catch a cold or other illness would do well to mince some garlic cloves up and down them with a glass of warm water. That is usually the end of the problem.

CARTILAGE

The famous Cuban studies by Dr. Lane with shark cartilage may have been overstated, and those who did well in his study were taking other active treatments including Hoxsey formula. I have not been convinced that it is cost-effective, and have never prescribed it. Patients I have observed taking it have had little change.

- Cartilage is avascular - it contains no blood vessels, and does contain substances which inhibit angiogenesis.
- Shark cartilage may be useful, but quality and price issues have deterred its wide acceptance.
- Bovine tracheal cartilage preparation Catrix has produced dramatic improvement and even remissions in human cancers given by injection and then orally at 8 of 375 mg capsules every 8 hours.

SOY ISOFLAVONES

Soy foods are strongly associated with reduced risk of breast, prostate, and other hormone dependent cancers as well as lung cancer in smokers. Despite many good animal studies and technical papers on its mechanisms of action, there are no actual human clinical studies on its use as a therapy.

1. In the lab 45 mg stimulates breast cancer cell proliferation, higher doses inhibit breast cancer. In humans the effect is consistently inhibitory. Most important is the exposure to soy before menarche.
2. genestein is reported to inhibit angiogenesis, reduce estrogen levels, partly block estrogen receptors, inhibit topoisomerase II and enhance efficacy of radiotherapy.
3. soy isoflavones inhibit DNA gyrase and induce apoptosis
4. soy protease inhibitors help maintain cell contact inhibition and reduce tumor invasiveness.
5. Tofu increases sex hormone binding globulin and reduces the testosterone/estradiol ratio.
6. Fermented soy foods are more bioavailable and safer. Unfermented soy foods can inhibit the thyroid gland.
7. Soy isoflavones are incompatible with Tamoxifen therapy
8. The Chinese developed a nitrogenated low temperature fermented organic soy beverage Haelan in the early 1980's as a hospital nutrition suplement. It is extremely rich in the anti-cancer isoflavones:

    genistein 228 mcg/ml
    genistin 222 mcg/ml
    daidzein 184 mcg/ml

It is also high in protease inhibitors which reduce mutation in cancer cells. It is an excellent source of bioactive free amino acids (protein). The usual dose is 8 ounces daily.

DR. LOFFLER

Dr. Fred Loffler, N.D. treats cancer with dietary modification, to balance acid and alkaline. His sensible food combining diet removes refined foods and red meat. He supplements with chelated zinc 10 mg 3 times a day, and phosphoric acid drops (Standard Process Labs) to adjust the acid/alkaline balance (pH) of the patient. Dr. Loffler has practiced naturopathic medicine for over 50 years.

BROMELAIN

A protein digesting enzyme extracted from pineapple stems. Better quality products will state a rating of their protein-busting activity from actual bioassays. For example, a GDU of 4 means 1 milligram of this bromelain product will liquefy 4 milligrams of animal gelatin.
1. reduces metastases by modulating cell adhesion
2. alters cytokine levels
3. fibrinolytic
4. reduces platelet aggregation
5. increases absorption of some medications, particularly water-insoluble bioflavenoids such as quercitin.

KELLEY METABOLIC CURE

William Kelley, MS, DDS cured himself of pancreatic cancer in 1964 with a program based on a raw food diet, supplements, coffee enemas, liver flushes and pancreatic enzymes.   The combination of pancreatic enzymes is claimed to 'destroy and strip away about 97% of such starch capsules, thereby enabling tumors to be recognized, digested, liquefied and removed from person's bodies via their bloodstreams.' This is the rationale behind the popular *Mugos Wobenzyme* products.

The use of pancreatic enzymes for cancer originated in 1902 with John Beard, an embryologist at the University of Edinburgh. Later Drs. Ernst Krebs & Ernst Krebs Jr. revived the enzyme concept, combining it with laetrile.   The Kelly program will trigger an initial rise in tumor markers, and the tumors may swell. The white blood cell count will rise, and as the tumors are breaking down the patient will experience flu-like achiness, fever, headache, nausea, and irritability. The program is given in 25 day cycles with 5 days rest between cycles to allow elimination of tumor wastes. High response rates are claimed in his books *Cancer Cure* and *Cancer - Curing the Incurable.*

Recall Pottinger's theory that solid tumors arise in sympathetic dominant cases which have low pancreatic enzymes. Nicholas Gonzalez practices a variant of the Kelly protocol, giving sympathetic dominant types a vegetarian diet with large doses of B-complex vitamins, magnesium and potassium; these folks need lots of vigorous aerobic exercise and pancreatic enzymes. For the parasympathetic dominant types with immune cell cancers such as leukemia and lymphoma he prescribes high intake of red meat, large doses of calcium, zinc, selenium, vitamin B12 and pantothenic acid - but avoids magnesium, potassium, thiamine, riboflavin and niacin.

Dr. Gonzalez also routinely uses coffee enemas and glandular remedies.

Doses of proteolytic enzymes range to 40 capsules daily.

BASIC CANCER THERAPY DIET

1. Reduce processed and canned foods.

2. Increase fresh foods, especially organic vegetables. Raw foods are alive, energizing and healing. The best foods are ones which you could have picked or gathered in nature, as your ancestors did.

3. Protein: 25-30% of calories. Avoid grain or silage fed red meats; substitute wild game, organic meat, fresh wild fish and seafood, organic poultry, whey, eggs, fresh nuts and fermented soy products. If hard to digest acidify gut & consider plant-source protease enzymes and betaine hydrochloride supplements. Eat food your ancestors could have hunted, fished or milked.

4. Choose cultured, soured and organic milk products.

5. Reduce sugar intake, and minimize wheat and starchy vegetables.

6. Fats: 20-30% of calories. Cook with extra virgin grade olive oil; Flax oil, sesame oil, evening primrose oil or fish oil may be supplemented. Other acceptable oils include cold-pressed canola, peanut, or sunflower. Butter is permitted.

7. Increase omega 3 fats EPA and DHA as in fish, cod liver oil or seal oil. Nuts like almonds and walnuts are a source of very good fats, as are seeds such as sesame, flaxseed, pumpkin and sunflower.

8. Reduce omega 6 fats, trans-fatty acids and arachidonic acid as in corn oil, margarine, shortening, and hydrogenated fats.

9. Pure water, green tea, rooibos tea and taheebo tea

10. Starches: 40 - 55% of calories. Emphasize legumes (peas & beans), soy, broccoli, carrot, celery, onion, garlic, squash, parsley, sprouts, tomato, beets, dark leafy greens, whole grain rice, rye and millet. Fresh juices - carrot, beet, parsley, and greens such as wheat grass.

11. Consider supplements of antioxidants vitamins. A, C, E, carotenes, selenium, chlorophyll, fiber.

Chapter Five - BOTANICALS & PLANT EXTRACTS IN CANCER CARE

Many plants have shown anti-cancer properties against cancer cells in test tubes *in vitro* and in living creatures *in vivo*, but only a few have been developed further. Highly cytotoxic extracts, such as the alkaloids from periwinkle and the etopisides from *Podophyllum*, have occasionally been made into patented drug isolates or synthetics, crossing over into orthodox medicine. Plants are biological entities, living beings, with many survival needs in common with us. They have DNA, so cytotoxic anti-DNA compounds are uncommon. Plants have almost unimaginably varied and subtle mechanisms for modulating biochemical systems. Many traditional plant medicines are treasure troves of potent but relatively non-toxic biological modifiers.

Whole plant extracts are not patentable as drugs, and are more difficult to fit into drug-style blinded studies. The elaborate formulae of Traditional Chinese Medicine, coupled with the TCM revulsion for placebo, has caused many time-proven cancer remedies to be ignored by Western medicine. Despite being used rationally by millions of doctors on billions of people for thousands of years, the white coat crowd still considers them completely "unproven". The "scientific" doctor can put people on long-term drug therapy with a synthetic drug which may have been given to humans for as short a time as 4 to 6 weeks in a drug trial, and they will tell you they know what it will do to you. That is quite remarkable - they must be psychic! How many drugs have been recalled or faded from use when long term harm or unexpected adverse affects show up after some years of this crude human experimentation?

Still, the same brain trust will tell you ginseng is potentially dangerous because "we don't know what it will do". I always say a physician's job is to *manage risk, not just avoid risk*. If they don't know it is safe after millenia of use, prove it isn't or step aside. The Hoxsey Formula, Essiac, and many other botanical approaches from European, Native American and Eclectic herbology are being used today without benefit of any scientific human studies. Many other promising herbs await screening. I am not so naïve that I trust the government, medical institutions and scientific community to scrutinize the home-spun remedies and sort out the good from the false, and develop the good ones into cures for us. Drug company pirates are exploiting traditional knowledge bases, stealing biological organisms, patenting them to exclude those who own them by heritage from further access, and converting them to synthetic commodities for resale at inflated prices. I inherited my genetics from my ancestors, not Monsanto. Their knowledge is my culture. I am free to access the God-given gifts for healing from the world around me and from within my own body and spirit. This is my inalienable right. Medicinal plants are part of my web of life.

HOXSEY FORMULA

Harry M. Hoxsey, ND (1901 - 1974) treated cancer with topical agents and an internal herbal formula said to have been used in the veterinary practice of his great-grandfather since 1840. Horses with cancer were apparently cured by extracts of the herbs applied as a salve. Similar formulas are found in the textbook of Dr. Eli Jones, MD - an American homeopath and herbalist who was famous for his work in cancer at the turn of the Twentieth Century. A very similar formula called Syrup Trifolium Compound was developed by Parke-Davis & Company in 1890. Extract of Trifolium Compound was a variation listed in the 1898 edition of King's American Dispensatory. Compound Fluid Extract of Trifolium was a recognized remedy in the 1926 National Formulary. It was widely used by many physicians.

Harry Hoxsey was a home-spun legend, who had flamboyant style, and was controversial, yet achieved legal and peer recognition for being able to cure cancer. Two USA federal courts upheld the therapeutic value of the tonic, and the American Medical Association admitted that the external salve had merit. Harry wrote a book describing his methods titled *You Don't Have to Die*. The failed attempt by Dr. Malcolm Harris, Secretary of the AMA to buy the secret tonic formula - for his own profit - resulted in years of harassment and arrests. Harry won a major settlement in a defamation lawsuit over a description of him as a "quack feeding off the flesh of the dead and the dying" and the lie that his father's death resulted from cancer, when in fact it he died from the infection erysipelas. Through various manipulations, including making naturopathy illegal in Texas, site of his largest clinic, he was driven from the field, without any scientific investigation of his claims. Harry closed up his clinics in the USA in the late 1950's. His former head nurse Mildred Nelson continued his clinical style in Tijuana, Mexico as the Biomedical Clinic, since 1963. Harry died in 1974, ironically of prostate cancer. His fascinating and politically charged career was documented in the 1987 film *Hoxsey - Quack Who Cures Cancer? - How Healing Becomes a Crime*.

Hoxsey stated that cancer developed as a result of -
1. low cellular potassium ions
2. poor thyroid function
3. poor liver function
4. poor elimination of toxins

Hoxsey may have had a mail-order degree, and may have been unsophisticated, but he had a clear concept of cancer as a disease resulting from a disturbance of the entire internal ecology and metabolism. He viewed his herbal extract as a *tonic* which was *alterative*, meaning it cleansed and strengthened all the vital organs.

Only the topical powders and salves applied to burn off tumors were viewed by Hoxsey as directly "anti-cancer" medications. His view of cancer as a constitutional and blood disease is typical of the Eclectic viewpoint as espoused by Eli Jones, and by naturopathic physicians today.

The Hoxsey cancer clinics used a secret herbal tonic of alcohol-free fluid extracts made from fresh herbs. It was independently analyzed to contain, per 5 ml:

20 mg red clover blossom	*Trifolium pratense*
20 mg licorice root	*Glycyrrhiza glabra*
20 mg burdock root	*Arctium lappa*
20 mg buckthorn bark	*Rhamnus frangula*
10 mg queen's root	*Stillingia sylvatica*
10 mg Oregon grape root	*Berberis aquifolium*
10 mg poke root	*Phytolacca decandra*
5 mg Honduras bark	*Cascara amarga*
5 mg prickly ash bark	*Xanthoxylum flaxineum*
150 mg potassium iodine	KI
U.S.P. Aromatic elixir 14	flavoring syrup

Some speculate that mayapple *Podophyllum pelatrum* may have been a constituent as well. This toxic herb later gave rise to the drug Etoposide, now in use in regular medical oncology.

The tonic was diluted by putting 2 fluid ounces in 14 ounces of tap water. Adult dose was 1 to 5 teaspoonfuls 4 times daily after meals and at bedtime. For children the dose was 5 to 30 drops 4 times daily. The tonic was often prescribed for 5 years, then to be taken for 3 to 4 months every Spring and Fall. Reactions such as a rash on the forehead, face or neck, frontal headaches, discharges and bowel intolerance may occur, necessitating a reduced dosage until cleared. This is likely due to the potassium iodide. Most patients tolerate it very well.

The patient was also given dietary restrictions, including the strict avoidance of tomatoes, pork, salt, vinegar, alcohol, sugar, white flour and processed foods. Patients were advised to drink lots of pure water, and juices such as unsweetened grape juice.

Hoxsey claimed a cure rate of 25% for internal cancers, and up to 60% for breast cancer.

Hoxsey claimed a cure rate of 85% for skin and external cancers, which he treated with *escharotics* - salves which kill cells on contact and cause a layer of tissue to dissolve and slough off. Open wounds were dusted with boric acid as a disinfectant.

Hoxsey Red Paste - combines zinc chloride, antimony trisulphide, and bloodroot *Sanguinaria canadensis* powder. This caustic and cytotoxic paste is painful, killing all tissue it contacts. It is very useful on melanomas.

Hoxsey Yellow Powder - combines USP Sulphur 2 oz, arsenic sulphide 0.5 oz, and 6 oz talc. Grind for a full hour in a mortar to solubilize. It only kills cancer cells. It is also very painful.

A healing ointment of Vaseline, rosin, refined camphor, beeswax, tincture of myrrh *Commiphora abyssinica*, and oil of spike – spikenard or *Aralia racemosa?* was used to aid any damaged non-cancerous tissue.

Red clover blossom *Trifolium* boiled down to a tarry solid extract which was applied topically, sometimes with the addition of *Sanguinaria* extract.

Phytolacca F.E. (fluid extract) 1:16 dilution as a compress was put on breast tumors for 4 weeks, and would promote drainage and even expulsion of the tumors through the skin. The cancer can literally come to the surface and fall right off.

Dr. Steve Austin, ND has observed that the Biomedical Center in Tijuana, Mexico is having moderate success salvaging perhaps 20% of a variety of advanced, medically terminal cases. Results of an informal and limited follow-up study were published in 1984. Mildred Nelson estimates 80% of cases respond to the therapy.
A recent investigation of the Hoxsey method by the University of British Columbia was "inconclusive", citing a lack of "sufficient time, personnel and funds".
Thanks for nothing! My own experience is similar to Dr. Austin's, seeing occcassionally dramatic results in astrocytoma, lymphoma, breast cancer, etc. I have often combined the *Red Clover Combination* from St. Francis Herb Farm in Cormack, Ontario, with homeopathic remedies such as *Conium, Carcinosum, Arsenicum* and Pascoe nosodes such as *Gliom, Lymphangitis* or *Prostata.* I prescribe one dropperful (20 to 25 drops) three times daily, in a little water, sip slowly, take no food or drink for 15 minutes. I do not use it in all cases, and I would not stake my life on it alone, but it is a reasonable adjunct in selected cases.

ESSIAC

Essiac was named by the Canadian public health nurse Rene Caisse, who learned of the formula in 1921. Rene met a patient who attributed her survival of breast cancer to a herbal mix originating with Ojibway First Nations. It is a decoction (water extraction) of:

Sheep sorrel	*Rumex acetosella L.*
Slippery elm bark	*Ulmus fulva*
Burdock root	*Arctium lappa*
Indian rhubarb root	*Rheum officinalis*

The popular brand *Flor-Essence* adds watercress herb, kelp, blessed thistle and red clover to the traditional, and some would say authentic Essiac formula.

Respirin Corporation owns the rights to the original Essiac formula and trade name, yet others claim variations that are the "real McCoy".

Like the Hoxsey formula, this mixture is a rich source of anthraquinones emodin and rhein which stimulate PGE2 synthesis, alter calcium transport, are antiinflammatory, antitumor and antibacterial. Caisse had many anecdotes to tell, and had some medical referrals of cases, but scientific testing on animals at the National Institutes of Health (NIH) in Bethesda, Maryland was inconclusive, and the therapy nearly passed into history on her death. It was repopularized recently by Elaine Alexander after a CBC radio program on Rene Caisse's life.

A standardized and authentic formula is made by Resperin Canada, who obtained the rights to her formula in 1978, just before Rene passed on.

The well respected naturopathic oncologist Dr. Jim Chan, N.D. has seen varied responses, the best results being in patients who have not had extensive chemotherapy or radiation. Unfortunately for Jim and I, few patients we see in British Columbia fall into this category.

This herbal formula is healthful, keeps the bowels moving, but is not in my experience and opinion a primary stand-alone cancer therapy.

ONCOLYN

Oncolyn is a proprietary combination of polyphenols and anthocyanins developed by Dr. Arthur Djang, M.D., Ph.D., M.P.H. Dr. Djang was a prominent orthodox medical researcher who pioneered the ninhydrin technique of latent fingerprinting, the isoenzyme technique for early diagnosis of myocardial infarction, and has many scientific publications in medical and cancer research. On retiring, he travelled to China, his ancestral homeland, where he was exposed to hospitals integrating Western allopathic and Eastern TCM methods.

He returned with some ideas for natural anti-cancer formulations, which he verified with cell culture and animal research techniques.

The Oncolyn formula is not published, so I do not know what it contains. My investigation suggests green tea polyphenol extract and grapeseed extract may be present, and one source suggests it may also contain a seed extract, perhaps from apples. I wish I knew exactly. It is unethical for me to prescribe secret formulas.

Oncolyn has been shown in tissue culture and rodents to be antioxidant, dismutagenic, pro-differentiation, anti-angiogenic, and anti-metastatic. Dr. Djang says 1 tablet daily will neutralize the toxins of tobacco smoking. For cancer the prescribed dose is 1 tablet with 500 mg vitamin C, 3 times daily before each meal,
and vitamin E 400 I.U. twice daily.   Improvement is expected in about 2 weeks.
 I have observed a number of significant responses to this product, for example two cases of advanced pleural mesothelioma which made a dramatic regression. That is a tough cancer to treat by any means, so I was impressed.

It is unfortunate the formula is secret, but a conversation with Dr. Djang after a public lecture about his research did reinforce my committment to using green tea and grapeseed extracts. A combination of bioflavenoids and polyphenols had already become a core part of my basic cancer program, based on my experience and that of other naturopathic doctors. I like to add in curcumin and other synergists.

GREEN TEA

Unfermented green tea *Camellia sinensis* leaf is a source of polyphenols such as epigallocatechin-3-gallate (EGCG), epigallocatechin (EGC) and epicatechin-3-gallate (ECG). The top leaves are steamed to inactivate enzymes which would oxidize the polyphenols into tannins, as found in "black tea". Many large-scale epidemiology studies show a significant preventative value, particularly at intakes of 5 to 10 cups of tea daily. However, that is a lot of fluid, and too much caffeine for many people. Black tea ranges up to 80 mg of caffeine per cup, and green tea is less, but yields at least 10 mg per cup. Other stimulating alkaloids in the tea leaf are theobromine and theophylline. Certainly the capsulated standardized extract is more convenient to reach the doses needed to use it as a therapy, without excessive caffeine.

- It is known to inhibit many cancers, by blocking cells in G0-G1 phase and arresting cells in G2-M phase of the cell cycle
- Induction of apoptosis is dose dependent.
- Enhances wild type p53 expression.
- Inhibits oncogene expression.
- Inhibits protein kinase C activation by tumor promoters.
- Anti-angiogenic, strongly inhibits vascular endothelial growth factor induction.
- Inhibits IGF-1
- Anti-cachexic, inhibits TNF alpha (cachectin) as a primary polyphenol effect.
- Tea polyphenols are matrix protease inhibitors, inhibiting tumor spread.
- Inhibits topoisomerase I, an enzyme which plays a critical role in DNA metabolism and structure, making it essential for tumor cell survival. Effective drugs which inhibit this enzyme are limited by toxicity.
- Inhibits 5-alpha-reductase, reducing testosterone levels.
- The unique amino acid theanine increases Adriamycin uptake by tumors, significantly increasing therapeutic efficacy.
- Synergistic with curcumin.
- Reduces risk of cancer recurrence 50% in post-op stage I & II breast cancer.
- Shown to inhibit breast, colon, prostate, lung, esophageal, stomach, pancreas, urinary bladder and melanoma cancers.
- EGCG inhibits urokinase (uPA), an enzyme involved in tumor invasion and metastasis, via breaking down of the basement membrane cell junctions. uPA is over-expressed in most cancers.
- Catechins in green tea rapidly transfer electrons or hydrogen from ROS damage sites on DNA, preventing the development of strand breaks.

- Green tea polyphenols reduce DNA damage from ultraviolet radiation UV-A and UV-B, reducing the inflammation, erythema, and skin cell hyper- proliferation. Thus it prevents skin cancer and will reduce the growth of established tumors in the skin.

The tea leaf contains 8 to 12% polyphenol antioxidants, and 1 to 4% caffeine. A cup of brewed green tea yields 10 to 40 mg caffeine. For therapy one would need to drink several cups daily. Brew a better tea using water at a temperature below a hard boil. The limit is what the Chinese call "crab-eyes" size bubbles in the kettle - bigger than "shrimp-eyes" but smaller than "fish-eyes" size. A cool overnight infusion of two tablespoons green tea in a litre of room temperature water is also fine for medicinal use, if the caffeine intake is tolerable.

I like to use 1,500 mg daily of 95% polyphenol extract of green tea.

IMPORTANT NOTE: green tea polyphenol extracts deplete the blood of vitamin E, so always supplement this vitamin when using high doses of the extract.

Green tea is an excellent example of the new botanical strategies for cancer developed by researchers such as John Boik, who has a Masters degree in Oriental Medicine. Boik has found there is a lot of good information on the mechanisms of many herbs, and many animal studies showing anti-cancer properties, but when the dose is scaled up to human levels, they are impractical as medications. The TCM approach is to use complex formulations with several herbs, relying on *synergies* - positive interactions which amplify the effects several fold. Indeed, many new formulae depend on these combinations doing more than one could predict from just adding together the actions seen in single agent studies. The fabulous news is there are excellent synergies being noted clinically when some simple, cheap and safe plant extracts are combined. The downside is that multicomponent medications are more difficult to evaluate by scientific protocols which were developed to test single chemical drugs expected to have huge toxicity issues. Add in the politics and economics of science and medicine, and we have a situation were some excellent therapies are languishing without research funds to evaluate them. No published double blind human trials means most doctors feel ethically restrained from using them, and therefore the majority of cancer patients are stuck with "evidence-based" drug therapies proven to a high standard to be toxic and of very limited value.

ROIBOOS TEA

Roiboos or Red Bush tea comes from South Africa, and it is a very pleasant tasting tea which is extraordinarily antioxidant. It is also great to drink cold in the summer. While not proven to fight cancer, it seems healthful and adds flavor and variety.

GRAPESEED EXTRACT

Oligomeric-proanthocyanidins (OPC) in grape skins and seeds are powerful antioxidants, perhaps 50 times that of vitamin C and 20 times that of vitamin E. They are highly chemoprotective, and have significant effects on the vascular endothelium. OPC from pine bark was brought to Canada by Dr. Allen Tyler, ND, MD by way of the French scientist Professor Jacques Masquelier, who investigated its use by Quebec First Nations people. Chinese research has shown this antioxidant to be a balanced cancer treatment. OPC are significantly cytotoxic to human breast, lung and gastric adenocarcinomas, while at the same time enhancing the growth and viability of normal cells. OPC can regulate cell cycle/apoptosis genes p53, bcl2, and c-myc. OPC increase expression of Bcl-2 gene and reduce expression of p53 and c-myc genes. This is how they reduce healthy cell apoptosis caused by chemotherapy drugs, reducing their toxicity. The daily dose should be 200 mg or more.

Similar compounds are found in the TCM herb *Polygonum cuspidatum.*

 I have taken 200 mg of pine bark, bilberry or grapeseed OPC daily for over a decade. I consider it a critically important supplement for good health. OPC are also a staple treatment for chronic fatigue syndrome, stroke or brain injury recovery, and many other conditions. I do not believe the concept that some herbalists put forward that OPC enhance metastasis simply because they are a circulation enhancer.

BILBERRY

Vaccinium myrtillus or bilberry is a relative of the blueberry, cranberry and huckleberry. It is rich in anthocyanosides which are known to strengthen collagen. The anthocyanidin *delphinidin* in bilberry is a very powerful redox recycler of glutathione. Daily dose should be over 100 mg of an extract standardized to 25 to 37% anthocyanosides. Anthocyanidins combined with glutathione in the product *Recancostat* has been found to suppress advanced chemo-resistant colon carcinoma, with increased survival and weight gain.

CURCUMIN

Curcumin is derived from the yellow curry spice tumeric *Curcuma longa* or *yu jin*. Dietary intake is protective from various cancers.

- induces apoptosis in cancers eg liver, kidney, sarcoma & colon
- highly chemoprotective, blocks tumor induction by chemical carcinogens
- decreases interleukins to strongly reduce inflammation
- stimulates the reticulo-endothelial immune system
- activates phagocytosis
- inhibits complement pathways
- inhibits spontaneous DNA damage from lipid peroxidation
- induces heat shock protein hsp70 to protect cells from stress
- inhibits cancer initiation, promotion and progression
- significantly inhibits angiogenesis
- significantly inhibits number and volume of tumors
- reverses liver damage from fungal aflatoxins
- reduces mutagens in tobacco smokers
- combines well with genestein from soy
- synergistic with EGCG from green tea

Naturopathic physicians in the U.S.A. are using Vital Nutrients brand *BCQ* curcumin, bromelain and quercitin, 2 capsules 3 times daily. Canadian doctors use professional labels such as Advanced Orthomolecular Research (AOR) brand or Vitazan brand quercitin at 500 to 1000 mg 3 times daily.

BOSWELLIA

Boswellia serrata or Frankincense is a respected herb used for 5,000 years in Egypt, China and India. This gummy tree resin was a gift from the three wise men from the East (Magi) to the Christ-Child in the Christmas legend. It has always been prized as a pain reliever and natural anti-inflammatory, and was indeed a treasure of the ancient world and a gift fit for a King. Today we often use as a 65% extract of boswellic acid at 500 mg three times daily for pain and inflammation. Remember inflammation in late stage cancer is a slippery slope to disaster, so always have an anti-inflammatory component in the program.

- Inhibits lipoxygenase and 5-HETE eicosanoids
- Reduces activity of plasma betaglucoronidase and GAG synthesis
- Inhibits topoisomerase I & II better than campothecin or etoposide drugs.
- Studied in brain and nasopharngeal cancers and in leukemia. For example it reduces edema in brain cancers, reducing pressure inside the skull.

ALOE VERA

This succulent has acemannan polysaccharides in its leaf which are immune stimulating, thymus stimulating, increase antibody-dependent cytotoxicity, and inhibit angiogenesis. Aloe emodin is antimetastatic. Aloe reduces PGE2, inhibits kinins, histamine and platelet aggregation. Aloe root or cape aloe has a long history of use as a healer of gastro-intestinal (GI) ulceration and inflammation, and it relieves constipation. It is mandatory in any GI cancer.

I have had a number of very dramatic responses to an old formula called #42's in patients in great pain and on morphine who have become constipated and ill with no appetite. #42's are made of equal parts wormwood *Artemesia vulgaris* or *A. annua* tops and cape aloe *Aloe capensis* root powder, and the usual dose is 2 capsules 3 times daily or as needed. It is remarkable how little pain they have when their bowels move, and how their entire health picks up. This has rescued a number of patients from premature death, or death without awareness due to being mentally "snowed under" by opiates.

RED CLOVER BLOSSOMS

Trifolium pratense or red clover is a common ingredient in many herbal cancer formulas, including the Hoxsey Tonic. It contains the coumarin type phytoestrogens and tumor inhibiting compounds genistein, daidzein, biochanin and formononetin. Traditional herbalists call it a "blood purifier". Red clover tops contain significant levels of phytoestrogens as estriols, which are mild and can counteract the more cancer stimulating estradiols, perhaps by occupying the estrogen receptors, without triggering the same signals into the nucleus. The National Cancer Institute tested red clover 94 times, with only one slightly positive test showing insignificant activity against cancer. If it is useful, it is as an *alterative* as described by the Eclectic herbalists: normalizing circulation, assisting digestion, accelerating eliminative processes, thus correcting faulty metabolism.

WORMWOOD

Artemisia vulgaris or absinthum is a traditional medicine for parasites, including malaria. It is very useful in cancer as #42 capsules described above. It relieves constipation, even severe cases bound up by morphine type drugs taken for pain - and as an added bonus, relieves pain by detoxifying. Furthermore, by removing parasites the level of inflammatory cytokine growth promoters is reduced.

GRAVIOLA

Annona muricata is also called graviola, soursop, and paw paw. It is a small evergreen tree with large glossy leaves, native to tropical America from the Caribbean to the Amazon. Its large heart shaped edible fruit is slightly sour and acid, and it is widely used in drinks and sherbets. Graviola leaves have long been used in local folk medicine for diarrhea, as a lactogogue to increase breast milk, for viral and bacterial fevers and for worms and parasites. Its seeds are crushed to make a stronger remedy for worms and parasites, and are strongly insecticidal. The leaves and bark are used indigenously for diabetes, heart disease, asthma, hypertension, in difficult childbirth, influenza and cough. In general it is cooling, sedative and antispasmodic. Among its many constituents are procyanidin, P-coumaric acid, beta-sitosterol, stigmasterol, myristic acid, HCN, malic acid, and unique *acetogens*.

In 1976 the National Cancer Institute found the acetogenins to be definitely cytotoxic to cancer cells. The most potent acetogenins have adjacent bis-tetrahydrofuran rings (THF), e.g. bullatacin. The mechanism of cytotoxicity is inhibition of mitochondrial Complex I electron transport, robbing the cells of ATP energy. In tumor cells they also inhibit the NADH oxidase of plasma membranes, which with ATP depletion thwarts energy dependent resistance mechanisms.

Graviola is active against breast, colon, pancreatic, prostate and other cancer cells *in vitro*. One test reported its activity in such a screening test to be thousands of times more potent than the common chemotherapy drug Adriamycin. No blinded human studies have been reported. It is clearly safe to use, is immune building, antibacterial, antiviral and antiparasitic, and is tonifying. The usual dose is 2 to 5 grams twice daily of the powdered leaf, 1 to 3 ml twice daily of a 4:1 tincture, or ½ cup 1 to 3 times daily of a tea of the leaf or bark.

ASHWAGANDHA

Withania somnifera - ashwagandha or winter cherry is a herb from the Hindu Ayurvedic tradition. Think of it as the East Indian equivalent of ginseng. It is an adaptogen, helping the body deal with stress. It is a slightly sedative nervine, antioxidant, immune modulating, blood-building and rejuvenating. Ashwagandha prevents loss of adrenal gland function, vitamin C, and body weight when under stress. It increases function in the dopaminergic systems. Ashwagandha is anti-inflammatory, via inhibition of cycloxygenase. It is quite non-toxic even with long-term use.

Ashwagandha is a great protectant from the damage to healthy cells by chemotherapy and radiation. It particularly protects bone marrow from damage, and stimulates stem cell proliferation to replace red blood cells, white blood cells and platelets. It also enhances therapeutic effectiveness of radiation against cancer cells because of an anti-tumor and radiosensitizing steroidal lactone *withaferin*.

MISTLETOE

Viscum album or *sang ji sheng* is a hemiparasitic plant which has subtle variations in its lectins depending on which species of tree it grows on i.e. fir, apple or pine. It is an immunological therapy for cancer which stimulates macrophages, T-cells, NK cells and cytotoxic complement. Injections increase cytokines TNFa, IL-1, Il-2, IL-5, IL-6, GM-CSF, gamma interferon and others. The anthroposophical product *Iscador* is my favorite. After some training and supervision most patients will self-administer every 1 to 3 days as a subcutaneous injection. A small dose is placed just under the skin to form a little bubble, which should provoke a red flare like an allergic hive or welt, as the immune system reacts. Inflammatory reactions are expected, and occasionally become problematic and require desensitization procedures. It is common to see tumor progression decelerate or even stop, improved general health, and reduced pain. It is a good bone marrow stimulant in drug-induced myelosuppression and in primary marrow diseases. The results I have seen in managing advanced cancers has been dramatic. Increased survival time in many advanced cancers is well documented in European studies. Quality of life is nearly always significantly improved.

It has amazed me, since my youthful days in cancer research, how North American doctors can ignore good science from Europe and other countries we normally think of as part of our Western civilization. The regional chauvinism is very strong, and many scientists here scoff at what I consider top science journals from Britain, Germany, etc. Unless their own Good Old Boys do the work in America with drug money, it is suspect. Those Germans and Brits do use herbs and homeopathics, they probably even use food as medicine, so they cannot be real scientists, can they? Chinese, Asian, African and other countries are also treated as if they are rank barbarians who cannot hold a test-tube right side up. Globalization has not reached medicine yet. I am proud to be able to offer "world medicine" to my patients.

"There are more things in heaven and earth than are dreamed of in your philosophy......"
Hamlet, William Shakespeare

The most High hath created medicines out of the earth, and a wise man will not abhor them.
Ecclesiasticus 38:4

CAT'S CLAW

Uncaria tomentosa or *Una de Gato* is a vine from Amazonia which indigenous tribes consider a sacred plant. Cat's claw inner bark contains pentacyclic oxindole alkaloids and carboxyl alkyl esters which are antioxidant and remarkably potent inhibitors of TNF-alpha synthesis. It may have a role in treating weight loss from cachexia and anorexia. It may reduce side effects of radiation therapy and chemotherapy – patients report less hair loss, nausea, skin problems and secondary infections. It has steroids and alkaloids with antibiotic, antifungal, antiviral and anti-allergy properties - in short, it is immune modulating. Peruvian traditional doctors are said to use it for cancers and other serious diseases, and since 1960 it has been used in some South American hospitals for cancer, with unconfirmed reports of 'consistent results'. James duke reports it is combined with curcumin and *Dracontium loretanum,* which is related to Jack-in-the-Pulpit. *In vitro* studies show 5 alkaloids with activity against lymphoma and leukemia cells. Use 1 ml of tincture or up to 2 grams of dry extract three times daily.

WHEAT GRASS JUICE

Ann Wigmore, N.D. emphatically recommends this juice, made fresh several times daily, consumed within 20 minutes of extraction. Chlorophyll has been emphasized as a cancer cure by our elders such as Dr. Fred Loffler, and Dr. Allen Tyler.

BROMELAIN

This protein digesting enzyme is commonly derived from pineapple stems. It is well documented to prevent clots by activating plasminogen, and may digest fibrin in clots once they have formed. It is definitely anti-inflammatory by depleting kininogen and also by activating series1 prostaglandins. It is an important adjunct to bioflavenoids such as quercitin and coenzyme Q10, which are otherwise quite poorly absorbed. It is a constituent of the popular proprietary European enzyme formula Wobenzym.

- reduces metastases
- modulates cell adhesion
- alters cytokine levels
- reduces platelet aggregation
- fibrinolytic
- antiinflammatory
- increases uptake of some drugs

LAETRILE

Various seeds of pit fruit, such as peaches and apricots, were used for cancer by ancient Chinese, Egyptians, Greeks and Romans. Laetrile was isolated from apricot pits by Ernst Krebs, MD in the 1920's. His son, Dr. Ernest Krebs, Jr., separated a cyanogenic compound from the enzyme *emulsin*, thought to dissolve the protein of the cancerous cell. He felt giving these two components separately at short intervals eliminated the toxicity seen with the whole kernal extract. The theory behind the use of these cyanide compounds is that normal cells have an enzyme *rhodanase* which dispels hydrocyanic gas formed during digestion. Cancer cells lack this enzyme, and have higher than normal levels of the enzyme *betaglucoronidase*, which is very susceptible to hydrocyanic poisoning. The betaglucoronidase enzyme is associated with the evolution sexual reproduction, including the penetration of sperm into an egg, and is normally only found in the early embryonic stage of human life, called a trophoblast. Cancer cells are the only mature cells with this enzyme in appreciable amounts. The laetrile would therefore be non-toxic to normal cells, and selectively destroy the cancer cell, targeting its unique chemical ability to digest through barriers and spread.

Dr. Kanematsu Sugiura at Sloan-Kettering found laetrile inhibits tumor growth and significantly retards metastasic spread. Despite his reputation as a meticulous scientist, his work was denied and ignored.

The Contreras Clinic in Tijuana, Mexico used it for many years. Dr. Austin and I agree that the Contreras clinic does help cancer cases, but not noticeably better than orthodox oncology. Laetrile doesn't appear to be a miracle drug, but may be useful.

Laetrile is considered by some to be cytotoxic, presumably from the cyanide compound amygdalin. It can cause nausea, vomiting, headache and dizziness. There have been unsubstantiated reports of death from cyanide toxicity. The American Cancer Society considers it an example of the worst sort of cancer quackery. The historical record on Laetrile has been polarized and distorted. I do not know who to believe. What little science there is has been lost in a cloud of propaganda.

I have never used Laetrile, out of trepidation over its reported toxicity.
I always prefer to work with the least toxic approach. I cannot say I have ever met anyone who has tried authentic Laetrile. However, many cancer patients today self-medicate with 4 to 5 raw apricot pits daily, and some claim results.

MILK THISTLE

Silybum marianum or milk thistle is the gentlest and most effective healer of the liver.

- highly hepatoprotective from chemical damage, so is recommended for any patient undergoing chemotherapy. It will support liver function where there are liver mets or a primary cancer of the liver.
- inhibits tumor necrosis factors – the TNF group.
- directly inhibits IL-1a and IL-1b production, which mediate acute phase pro-inflammation response including T and B immune cell activation.
- inhibits EGF, which drives carcinoma growth.
- the component *silibinin* inhibits cancer cell growth by 48% and induces apoptosis to increase by a factor of 2.5
- Significantly reduces phospho-mitogen-activated protein kinase/extracellular signal-regulated protein kinase 1/2 (MAPK/ERK1/2) to inhibit growth. Up-regulates or increases stress-activated protein kinase/ jun NH(2) terminal kinase (SAPK/JNK1/2) and p38 mitogen-activated protein kinase (p38 MAPK) activation.
- slows prostate and skin cancer growth

COFFEE

Coffee contains caffeine and theophyllines which block PI-3 kinase enzyme crucial to cell growth. It may have anti-clotting properties. It has long been used in Mexican cancer clinics as a retention enema of 4 to 6 ounces of brewed coffee to relieve pain, presumably by flushing toxins out of the liver by increasing bile flow. This seems strange to some, but it has a long history of use in hospitals and medicine. It works.

TAHEEBO

Tabebuia avellanedae or *Pau d'Arco* inner bark and heartwood contains anthroquinones and napthoquinones such as *lapochol*. Taheebo has been used since 1960 at Santo Andre Hospital in South America on terminally ill cancer patients. Native folklore suggested that it might be useful for breast cancer, Hodgkin's lymphoma, leukemia, cancer pain, and to increase the blood cell counts. Taheebo is anti-neoplastic, acting directly against oncogenes. Health Canada advises it is completely harmless as a beverage, but has "no proven merit in treating cancer".
It is regarded as a treatment for overgrowth of the yeast Candida albicans, parasites, bacterial and virus infections. This would be expected to reduce inflammatory growth factors, which would slow cancer growth. The inner bark chips need to be boiled for about 15 minutes, then steeped another 15 minutes. Drink it freely. As a tincture, use 15 to 20 drop 2 to 3 times daily. Very high doses can cause nausea, vomiting, and prolonged bleeding time. Some patients tell me it really helped them.

CHAPPARAL

The creosote bush *Harrea divertica Coville* leaves and twigs contain nordihydroguaiaretic acid (NDGA). This powerful antioxidant removes glucose from the cancer cells, reducing their growth. It has a long history of use by Native American practitioners for rheumatism, arthritis, urethral complaints, lymphatic swellings, and for tissue repair. It was popularized by Jason Winters, who claims it is especially effective for melanoma. He often combined it with red clover and gotu kola. Large doses will commonly cause nausea, loss of appetite, stomach ache and vomiting.

Occasional acute toxic cholestatic hepatitis and jaundice has been reported with chapparal, sometimes resulting in fulminant liver failure requiring liver transplantation, or resulting in death. Clearly a herb to use with caution. However, Dr. John Bastyr, ND used it freely in his arthritis formula, with no problems.

CARNIVORA

The Venus fly-trap plant *Dionea muscipula* juice is treated to remove poisonous constituents, then mixed with alcohol and water to make the patented phytonutrient Carnivora. It is an immune modulator used by some American Presidents. According to Dr. Helmut Keller, microbes, viruses, parasites and tumors are rapidly reduced by the activation of helper T-cells and inhibition of suppressor T-cells. Carnivora makes protein kinases which block the production of tumor proteins, starving the cancer cells. Carnivora also balances autoimmune disorders. A standard protocol is 12 ml. diluted in 250 ml. normal saline given intravenously in a 4 hour drip. Doses can range from 30 to 100 ml daily in 500 ml saline by a 4 hour I.V. drip. For brain cancers dilute the product in 20% mannitol to carry it across the blood-brain barrier. The product may also be taken in water or tea 120 to 250 drops daily. For disease in the respiratory tract it may be inhaled via a cool-steam vaporizer. Sterile preparations may be injected subcutaneously 1 ml. twice daily or intramuscularly 2 ml twice daily. An extract may be encapsulated, and taken at doses of 1 to 2 of 125 mcg capsules up to four times a day. It can cause a fever and increased white blood cell count. As we have seen with graviola, Coley's toxins, and mistletoe, the immune system is challenged, the reticuloendothelial system responds, and all manner of infections, parasites, viruses and the malignant cells are robbed of energy and forced into apoptosis.

PODOPHYLLUM

Podophyllum pelatrum or Mayapple yields the irritating resin *podophyllin*. Tinctured to 25%, podophyllin can be used as an escharotic to remove superficial basal or squamous cell carcinoma. I use this in a formulation I developed which I call 'Wart Death' to remove benign growths. An extract of this plant has been made into the synthetic chemo drug Etoposide.

HORSE CHESTNUT TREE

Aesculus hippocastanum leaves contain active coumarins, anticoagulants, antioxidants, and the hemolytic saponin *escin*. Its favorable impact on vascular permeability is inhibited by cyclooxygenase inhibitors. Escin protects the integrity of the vascular basement membrane, inhibiting invasion and metastasis. Use intermittently, for 2 to 4 weeks at a stretch, as it is slightly toxic to the kidneys. We use it extensively for varicose veins and hemmorhoids, both topically and internally.

PLANT STEROLS & STEROLINS

Beta-sitosterols and sterolins were discovered in the traditional Hottentot medicinal plant *Hypoxis repari* by Dr. Patrick Bouic, Ph.D., an immunologist from South Africa. These common plant fats are extremely powerful modulators of the immune system.
I use them with omega 3 oils for all autoimmune diseases. 1 to 3 capsules of a professional quality extract such as Vitasan Beta-sitosterol mix will increase the adrenal hormone building block DHEA, which reduces circulating cortisol.
Sterols and sterolins will increase IL-2, IFN-gamma, activate NK and T-cytotoxic C8 cells to lyse cancer cells, reducing inflammation and immunosuppression.
It is to be considered in squamous cervical cancer because it is active against human papilloma virus, giving a remission rate of 50% for HPV infections.
Sterols appear to be most useful in lymphomas and leukemias.

BERBERINE

Oregon grape root - *Berberis* or *Mahonia aquifolium* contains the alkaloid berberine, which has a long use in Chinese and other medical traditions as a broad-spectrum antimicrobial and ant-inflammatory. Other herbs containing this alkaloid are coptis, andrographites, barberry *Berberis vulgaris* and golden seal root *Hydrastis canadensis*. All are used for infections, including parasites. These 'cold' herbs cool inflammation. Berberine is a potent herbal cytotoxic alkaloid which poisons DNA topoisomerases I and II. Its pharmacological profile is very similar to the natural drug Camptothecin, which is now being used for a variety of cancers. Berberine induces apoptosis in leukemias and carcinomas. It is also is an excellent free radical scavenger of singlet oxygen and the superoxide anion radical. It is antimutagenic by modulation of DNA transcription.

BOTANICALS DESERVING FURTHER INVESTIGATION

<u>Rattlesnake plantain</u>: *Goodyera pubescens* is a scarce rainforest Orchid used by natives in North America for ulcers and cancers. Many interesting testimonials are on file at the B.C. Cancer Research Centre, and my inquiries into some of these cases suggests real potential for external and internal use. The plant is rare, delicate, and not forageable.

<u>Bindweed</u>: *Convovulus arvensis L.* is a common field weed related to Morning-glory vines. Dr. Daniel Rubin, N.D. has found it has signifigant C-statin angiogenesis inhibitor properties.

<u>Graviola</u>: *Annona murica* was found to be very powerful but the active principles could not be made synthetically to produce a drug, so the research money dried up - or so the legend goes.

<u>*Saposhnikovia divericata:*</u> rhizhome has an acid arabingalactan polysaccharide Saposhnikovan A which is a potent potentiator of the reticulo-endothelial immune system.

<u>Pseudo-ginseng</u>: *Panax pseudoginseng var. notoginseng* because it moves stagnant blood but prevents hemorrhage.

<u>Violets</u>: *Viola papillonacea* – fresh violet leaves as infusion or a compress relieves pain and inhibits tumor growth. Used by Hippocrates and often mentioned by herbalists throughout the ages.

It is a fact of history that the source of many advances in orthodox medicine has been the botanical formularies of the irregular physicians, the homeopaths, and the herbal "wise women" and "wise men" of the world. Each time regular doctors falter, and the so-called war on cancer has indeed stalled, there are raids on the knowledge base of those on the front-lines of natural medicine. The originators of the clinical use of these valuable medicines are almost never acknowledged, for they are of course quacks for using them without the blessing of the science industry bio-pirates.

It seems as if until a God-given healing force on the planet is turned into a commodity for profit, it has no value in the current medical system. This must end. The healing power of nature has the same value as life. Without it, no medicine works.

Chapter Six - TRADITIONAL CHINESE MEDICINE (TCM) IN CANCER

The classic Eight Principles system of TCM categorizes patient's conditions and matches up herbs in terms of *hot/cold, excess/deficiency, yin/yang* and *interior/exterior*. Further consideration is given to the state of various forms of the vital energy chi or qi, the state of the blood, the vital essences such as jing and parameters such as stagnancy, dampness, dryness, fire, wind, toxins, phlegm and obstructions. Once the language and cultural code is cracked, these are actually quite logical and simple rationales for selecting therapies. An experienced TCM practitioner will *always* be able to discern a strategy to improve balance and health, and can readily monitor through pulse and tongue diagnosis whether the overall state of the patient is improving or not.

CHI DEFICIENCY - use immunostimulants such as *Astragalus membranaceus* or huang qi, *Ligusticum porterii*, and licorice root. *Fuzheng peibeng* nourishing formulations like Bu Zhong YI Qi Wan reinforce the body essence to build a foundation of positive chi. Ginseng and Notoginseng extracts are immune stimulating. Immune tonics work best when given early in the day, such as one dose at breakfast and another before lunch.

STAGNANT BLOOD - induce fibrinolysis and inhibit platelet aggregation with cayenne *Capsicum frutescens*, horse chestnut *Aesculus hippocastanum*, carthamus flower *Carthamus tinctorius*, cordyalis rhizome *Cordyalis yanhusuo*, notoginseng *Panax* pseudoginseng and tumeric *Curcuma longa*. Protein and tyrosine kinase inhibitors in soy miso inhibits platelet aggregation. The Chinese use the term *huoxue huay* for enlivening the blood and dissolving stasis. Stagnancy from lack of chi flow makes tumors form.

YIN DEFICIENCY - nourish with ligusticum root *Ligusticum porterii*, lycium fruit *Lycium chinense*, Chinese foxglove root *Rehmannia glutinosa*. Avoid astragalus *Astragalus membranaceous* and atractylodes root *Atractylodes macrocephala*.

CLEAR HEAT TOXINS - inflammation or fire toxin are reduced by isatis root *Isatis tinctoria*, cassia *Cassia obtusifolia* and formulae like Qing Wen Bai Dou Yin. The Chinese term is *qingri jiedu* for clearing heat and eliminating toxins. Patients with a red base to the tongue covered with a thick yellow patchy coat are very hot and toxic!

DISPERSE MASSES - tumors accumulate when the chi or vital force fails to move matter and it stagnates and forms into hard masses. Herbs which soften and disperse these perform the function *ruanjian sanjie*.

DISPERSE CONGEALED PHLEGM - phlegm and dampness can obstruct channels and create tumors. Herbs which dissolve phlegm and disperse dampness perform the function *huatan qushi*.

POISON AGAINST POISON - toxic herbs can be used, similar to Western style cytotoxic chemotherapy, and this is called *yidu gongdu*. This strategy of *gong xie* means "attack the disease evil", and contrasts with the more common *fuzheng* supportive and corrective strategies.

Herb formulae used in cancer may have many ingredients, with groups or modules of herbs designed to serve one of these core principles of treatment, and with accessory herbs which direct the others to a particular organ or meridian. Each formula is customized to the individual condition, and not just to the disease. If one aspect of the condition improves before another, that cluster of herbs may be removed from the formula.In North America we may use pill forms of the formulae, and may use two or more different formulae together, each specific to one of the treatment principles.

MUSHROOM POLYSACCHARIDES

Asian traditional medicine has long used mushrooms such as *Coriolus versicolor*, maiitake *Grifola frondosa*, shitake *Lentius edodes* and reishi *Ganoderma lucidum* or *ling zhi* as immune stimulants. All can be effective if good quality extracts are used.

Reishi mushrooms contain cytotoxic triterpenes which have been shown to inhibit DNA synthesis via DNA polymerase beta. PSP and PSK are proprietary hot water extracts from fungal mycelia that run about 30% high molecular weight polysaccharides (HMWPS). They are proven immunomodulators via inhibition of cytokines IL-8 and TNFa. Coriolus PSK stimulates natural killer cells, lymphocytes to increase IL-2 by 2.5 fold. Trials with 1,500 mg twice daily have shown increased survival in patients undergoing chemotherapy with cisplatin for many cancers.

Shiitake lentinan corrects ovarian cancer resistance to cisplatin or 5-FU.

AHCC (active hexose correlated compound) is a proprietary Japanese low molecular weight compound from fermented shiitake and other medicinal mushrooms grown in rice bran, which has been found to prevent many chemo side-effects and increase the effectiveness of methotrexate, 5-fluorouracil and cyclophosphamide when used at doses of 3 grams daily. It may also protect from radiation damage and reduce stress from surgery. It is particularly useful in protecting chemo patients from damage to bone marrow, prevent hair loss, and has demonstrated it can reduce nausea, vomiting, pain and can improve appetite.

BU ZHONG YI QI TANG

Rich in HMWPS from *Lycium barbarum*, *Gynostemma pentaphyllum* or *jiao gu lan*, *Acanthopanax senticosus* or Siberian ginseng, and *Astragalus membranaceus*. Increases IL-2 and may be synergistic with melatonin and glutathione.

GINSENG

Panax ginseng or *ren shen* contains ginsenosides which are known to be antineoplastic -

- cytotoxic
- cause G1 arrest similar to p53 protein
- induce redifferentiation
- induce apoptosis.
- activate and modulate the reticulo-endothelial immune system
- activate p21 gene transcription, and expression of p27 protein.
- suppress Bcl-2, caspase 3, 5-alpha-reductase, androgen receptors, cell adhesion, invasion and metastasis.

Traditionally ginseng is used as a tonic for digestion and fatigue in the elderly, and as a panacea for longevity. It is proven to lower blood sugar by increasing insulin receptors, reduce stress reaction, and enhance immunity. It is believed to improve lassitude, pain tolerance, mental concentration, memory, physical vitality and appetite. The traditional style of use is a tea of ginseng root. This is a warming and digestive stimulating beverage. The root is made into the more *yang* energy "red" ginseng by repeated steaming. This neutralizes certain enzymes. Women are often given the "white" or unprocessed root, which is more *yin*. I put an inch or two of a stout root in a ceramic Chinese herb pot full of water, set inside a large double-boiler pot, at a low boil for a few hours. Ginseng alone or with royal jelly and other herbs is energizing and tonifying for yang and chi deficient patients. It may be synergistic with vitamin C for leukemia.

The patented natural product *Careseng* is an enriched extract with 8% Rh2 and 75% related aglycan ginsenosides which are synergistic. It is very potent, and strongly synergistic with cytotoxic compounds, activating execution caspases. It overcomes multidrug resistance (MDR gene) to restore tumor sensitivity in late-stage disease. It may block angiogenesis, and may block cancer cell entry into G1 growth phase, arresting tumor growth. A synthetic form of these ginsenosides is being developed as a drug under the designation PBD-2131.

PC SPES
A proprietary Chinese herbal formula for prostate cancer was manufactured by NovaSpes, Inc. Spes is Latin for "hope". Declared constituents included *Chrysanthenum rebescens*, *Isatis indigotica, Glycyrrhiza glabra, Ganoderma lucidum, Panax ginseng, Seronea repens, Scutellaria baicalensis, Panax notoginseng* (pseudoginseng). This formula was extremely potent, and had significant side-effects, as well as being very successful in treating prostate cancer. It would suppress androgen receptor expression as well as 5-alpha reductase. It induced apoptosis by down-regulating the genes bcl-2 and bcl-6, suppresses cell proliferation in a number of cancers in vitro, and acted as a radiosensitizer. Health Canada recently banned this product due to contamination with the drug Coumadin, a potent blood thinner, at doses equal to a low maintainence dose. Some batches also have been laced with diethylstilbesterol (DES) a very potent estrogen known to produce effects in users and in their offspring. I never used this product, as the side-effects were no better than the orthodox hormone blockade medications, and at much more cost. I had been burned before by Chinese products that looked "too good to be true". They usually turn out to be laced with drugs, as in this case. I have other Chinese herbs I trust which are quite a bit safer.

INTERNAL DISSOLUTION PILLS
This complex formula is very effective at shrinking a wide variety of cancers. It is rich, salty and somewhat difficult to digest, so may need adjunctive digestive support in delicate patients. It relieves pain, detoxifies and is anti-inflammatory.
Adults take 3 to 4 tablets 3 times daily after meals, with water.
Among its key ingredients are the Chinese classics for cancers: *peony root, ginseng, notoginseng, carthamus flowers, asari, scutellaria* and *cordyalis*. IDP's are very strong, may have a mutagenic componenet, and so are best used in short courses to aggressively shrink problem tumors, like a herbal blast of palliative radiation. I then try to hold the tumor in check with milder herbs during remissions.

ANTICANCERLIN
A TCM tablet for post-surgical long term management of carcinomas of the pancreas, stomach, rectum, liver and esophagus. It may also have a role in lung, urinary bladder, nasopharyngeal and thyroid cancers, as well as leukemia. It can shrink tumors, increase appetite and strength, relieve pain and reduce complications such as jaundice. In advanced pancreatic cancer the average remission is over 18 months.
Dose is 4 tablets (0.25 gram extract per tablet) 3 times daily. It is mild, safe, and cannot to be expected to do what some more aggressive formulas do. Add synergists.

PING XIAO PIAN

For solid tumors. *Alumen, Lacca Sinica Exsiccata* and *Guano Trogopterorum* disperse stagnation, activate the blood, which is antiinflammatory, analgesic and promotes tissue regeneration. *Strychni* seed stimulates the heart and nervous system to promote vital energy. *Agrimoniae* herb and *Aurantii* fruit are dispersive, cardiotonic, and stimulate digestion. *Sal Nitri* and *Curcumae* root complete the formula. A favorite of my colleague Dr. Geoff Szymanski, RAc, ND   A variation is sold to practitioners by Eden Herbs as *Can-Z*.

LIU WEI DI HUANG WAN

A classical formula for kidney yin deficiency.   For "false-fire" yin deficient patients, who show various inflammatory signs and symptoms. The key herb *Rehmannia glutinosa* tonifies the adrenal glands, prolongs the action of cortisol or the drug cortisone and antagonizes depression caused by steroid hormones. I have seen some wonderful remissions of cancer of the esophagus and stomach with this simple old formula. It heals and restores damaged kidneys too. For small cell lung cancer patients undergoing radiotherapy or chemotherapy it is shown to increase the proportion having a complete response, lengthen survival and reduce toxicity to blood elements. I give it in doses of 12 pellets twice daily of the patent medicine "Rehmannia Six".

LIU WEI HUA JIE TANG

This formula supplements qi, dramatically increasing long term survival in stomach cancer.

SHIH CHUAN DA BU WAN

Shiquan or "Ginseng & Tang kuei Ten Herb Formula" is a TCM formula containing *astragalus* and *ligusticum*. It has a long history of use to build the qi, blood, yin and yang - and since it builds all four of the vital elements, it is rightly called a supertonic. Shih chuan da bu wan is used in China for leukemia, stomach and uterine cancers. It has been shown to stimulate hemopoietic (blood-building) factors, and interleukin production. It can potentiate the effectiveness of chemotherapy drugs and reduce their toxicity, especially leukopenia, thrombocytopenia, weight loss and fatigue.

SHEN MAI ZHU SHE YE

Ginseng & Ophiopogon injectable fluid given at a dose of 50 ml. delivers 0.5 mg each of these herbs. Chinese research has shown superior results in reversing pancytopenia bone marrow suppression from chemotherapy drugs, compared to the Western drug Leucogen plus vitamins. The TCM strategy here is supplement original qi, boost the stomach qi, nourish the yin, engender fluids and clear heat.

JIN GUI SHEN QI

Supplements the kidney yang. Small cell lung cancer patients undergoing radiotherapy or chemotherapy have been given this formula with a positive increase in complete remissions, lengthened survival and reduced hemotological toxicity.

PISHEN FANG

Also called Juan Pi Yi Shen, this formula supplements qi and yang. It doubled survival in stomach cancer patients undergoing chemotherapy. Improvement was observed in body weight, appetite, increased macrophage activity, with reduced leukocytopenia, nausea and vomiting.

SHEN XUE TANG

This formula supplements the qi, yin, yang and blood. In stomach cancer treated by chemotherapy there was less diarrhea, vomiting and loss of appetite.

SI JUN ZI TANG

Used in China for medium stage liver cancer along with radiation therapy the 5 year survival rate is 43% - in USA the comparable survival rate is 6%. Builds qi, contains ginseng.

SHO-SAIKO-TO

A Japanese formulation of 7 Chinese herbs being tested at the Memorial Sloan-Kettering Cancer Center for ablation of non-resectable liver cancer (hepatocellular carcinoma). Phase 1 trials in Japan showed hepatoprotective, antiproliferative and immune-stimulating effects. This is a Kampo style standardized extraction of raw traditional herbs, prepared by Honso Pharmaceutical Co.

YI QI YANG YIN TANG

Treats esophageal and nasopharyngeal cancers in combination with radiation therapy. This formula supplements qi and yin, clears heat toxins.

YE QI SHENG XUE TANG

Supplements qi and blood, if given early in the day it supports DNA synthesis in the bone marrow, to reduce leukopenia. Sheng Xue Tang significantly improves immune indices like macrophage activity, T-helper lymphocyte counts, and NK cell function.

FU ZHENG SHENG JIN

For nasopharyngeal cancer in combination with radiotherapy. This formula supplements qi and yin, clears heat toxins.

YI KANG LING

Animal studies show tumor inhibition, low toxicity, immune stimulation, potentiation of cyclophosphamide and mitomycin.

FEI LIU PING

Supplements qi and clears heat toxins, used in primary bronchogenic carcinoma to support chemotherapy, it reduces toxicity and increases survival time.

LING ZHI FENG WANG JIANG

The reishi mushroom *Ganoderma lucidum*, "poor-man's ginseng" *Codonopsis pilosulae*, lychee fruit *Lycii chinensis*, and *Royal jelly*, the food of the Queen bee, and honey make up this pleasant and effective nutritive general tonic for the qi and blood. It greatly strengthens and invigorates the fatigued cachexic patient. It can restore appetite, nutrient and medication absorption and body weight. This is a real treasure. Take a vial (10 ml) every morning. If they are very Yang deficient combine this with true ginseng *Panax ginseng*, or Siberian ginseng *Eleutherococcus senticosus*.

SIBERIAN GINSENG

Eleutherococcus senticosus or *Acanthopanax senticosus* is a wonderful herb for fatigue and stress. It is not a true ginseng, but is an adaptogen herb from Northern China and Siberia which was used for purposes similar to the ginseng of Southern China. It balances blood sugar and is strengthening. I have taken it daily for many years. Siberian ginseng may inhibit sarcomas. Use *Wu Cha Seng* brand wild-crafted root, 4 tablets twice daily.

GOOSE BLOOD TABLETS

For lung, lymphatic or nasopharyngeal cancers.

JING WAN HONG OINTMENT

"Capital City Many Red Color" ointment treats radiation burns. It relieves pain promptly, decreases inflammation, reduces swelling, and detoxifies. It promotes regeneration and healing of burned tissue. The TCM mechanism is to Detoxify Fire Poison.

DANG GUI LU HUI

Effective formula for chronic myelocytic leukemia. The active principle appears to be indirubin in the *qing dai* or *Isatis tinctoria*, which is immune stimulating and inhibits DNA synthesis specifically in immature leukemic cells in the bone marrow. Synthetic indirubin is used at oral doses of 150-200 mg, is less toxic than the drug Myleran, but similar to hydroxyurea in GI toxicity, thrombocytopenia and marrow suppression.

YUN NAN BAI YAO

Yunnan Paiyao is an excellent formula of *Panax pseudoginseng var. notoginseng*. Called *san qi* in TCM, it may also be spelled Baiyao. It contains ginsenosides and also the unique saponin *notoginsenosides* or pseudoginsenosides protopanaxadiol and protopanaxatriol which distinguish it from ginseng. Extracts will scavenge superoxide radicals, contain antitumor polysaccharides, and are anticarcinogenic - but the herb is best known as a fantastic hemostatic.

- stops bleeding on contact or when taken internally. It will stop internal bleeding in the lungs, GI tract and nasopharyx from local cancers or from leukemia.
- relieves pain and stops swelling from blood stagnation
- corrects thrombocytopenia rapidly - platelets can double in just two weeks.
- Notoginseng has arabinogalactan polysaccharides which are potent stimulators of the reticulo-endothelial immune system.
- Notoginseng is a radiosensitizer, and has an anti-leukemic effect.

Use the powder directly on bleeding tissue. Take internally with water, 1 or 2 capsules or 0.25 to 0.50 grams (1/16 to 1/8 of the little glass bottle) of the loose powder. This powder was claimed to be a potent secret weapon of the Viet Cong because it saved many an isolated guerilla soldier by staunching bleeding from gunshot wounds or other trauma, when no medical assistance was available.

The Chinese use notoginseng unstintingly in many cancer formulations. It moves blood stagnation, or "cracks stagnant blood". This stagnancy causes the formation of all tumors. Stagnant blood also is said to be the cause of pain. This is what we naturopaths call a "crackerjack" herb for cancer.

FISH OTOLITH FORMULA

Specifically for brain or central nervous system (CNS) tumors. Such formulas rely on herbs which resolve blood stagnation and salty herbs to dissolve the masses. The kidneys rule the marrow, and they like their salt and blood.

ZHEN GAN XI FENG TANG

If the yang energy is agitated in cases of brain cancer, this mineral rich cooling formula will calm the patient and reduce seizures.

CAN JU TAN

Relieves headache, vomiting and other effects of brain cancers.

XIFENG RUANJIAN TANG

Extinguishes wind and softens accumulations, to dramatically increase survival with brain tumors. Scorpion, centipede and earthworms will seem strange to Westerners.

BUSHEN HUANTAN TANG

A simple all-plant formula which transforms phlegm and tonifies the kidney, and increases survival in brain cancer.

WEN DAN TANG

Transforms phlegm, rids dampness for brain tumor edema

PULMONARY TONIC TABLETS

Li Fei tablets treat the chronic dry cough in lung cancer patients with deficient lung yin, as does the syrup formula Qui Li Gao.

SALVIA

Sage *Salvia miltiorrhiza* or *dan shen* regulates the blood. It is synergistic with the COP chemotherapy protocol used in lymphoma.

POLYGONUM

Polygonum cuspidatum or *hu chang* is a herb rich in the anthraquinone emodin. It has been shown to significantly increase leukocyte counts in patients made leukopenic by radiotherapy.

BURDOCK ROOT

Burdock root *Arctium lappa* or *niu bang zi* contains lignans which reduce sex hormone bioavailability, induce differentiation, and inhibit tumor cell proliferation. John Boik suggests burdock seed tincture would be a useful synergist with the Hoxsey herbal formula. The Japanese eat it as "Gobi root".

SCUTE

Scutellaria baicalensis or *huang qin* normalizes platelet-induced hemostasis, associated with metastasis and tumor advancement. It is a Cox-2 inhibitor, which can assist in narcotic reduction and is also anti-inflammatory by inhibition of lipoxygenase. Several cytotoxic flavones have been identified. It has DNA binding activity, is anti-mutagenic, stimulates lymphocytes and white blood cells in general, inhibits conversion of fibrinogen to fibrin by thrombin, inhibits proliferation, inhibits protein tyrosine kinase, inhibits topoisomerase II, inhibits cAMP phosphodiesterase, decreases androgen receptor expression, and activates caspase-3 apoptotic enzymes. It is likely most useful in prostate, breast and vaginal cancers.

BUPLEURUM

Bupleurum chinense, Bupleurum falcatum or *chai hu* is a cooling herb used to treat liver qi stagnation. Its *saikosaponins* are strongly antiinflammatory, inhibit angiogenesis and induce apoptosis in liver cancer cells. The anti-inflammatory effect is due to stimulation of adrenal cortical trophic hormone (ACTH) from the pituitary gland, which in turn stimulates the adrenal gland to make more cortisol. The adrenal gland will actually increase in weight. Licorice is synergistic by reducing the breakdown of the cortisol produced.

The ancient formula Xiao Chai Hu Tang or "Minor Bupleurum Combination" is a classic for improving liver blood flow and function.

ISATIS

Isatis tinctoria or "dyer's woad" is the source of royal indigo purple dye. It is in the *Brassica* family and so contains anti-cancer *indoles*. It has beta-sitosterols which modulate the immune system. The leaves have an alkaloid *tryptanthrin* which is a strong COX-2 inhibitor, making it anti-inflammatory and anti-allergic. The root has traditionally been used for solid tumors and modern studies with the purified compound *indirubin* at 150 to 200 mg daily show responses in leukemia.

RUBIA

Rubia cordifolia or *qian cao gen* contains a peptide which strongly inhibits tumors in vivo.

CHINESE DIETETICS

Avoid beef, fatty meats, wine, goose, salt, excess sweets, and foods that are smoked, sour, fried, spicy, very rich or stimulating.

Mung bean sprouts and royal jelly are protective.

Foods are classified as hot, cold, yin, yang, and so forth, allowing diets to be formulated which balance and harmonize according to the Eight Principles diagnosis obtained by pulse and tongue assessment on each contact with the patient.

Chapter Seven -   ENERGY HEALING & OTHER REMEDIES

ACUPUNCTURE

Most people know acupuncture can relieve pain, even to the point where surgery can be done with little or no other anesthesia. However, when done in its proper context of traditional Chinese medicine (TCM) diagnosis and prescription, it can balance the parasympathetic and sympathetic branches of the autonomic system, reset the command and control centers in the central nervous system, and rebalance the entire organism. It reminds the various parts to reconnect and work together for the common good. This is so important in a disease such as cancer, which is all about a loss of control. Acupuncture needling causes the local release of platelet aggregation factor (PAF) and kinins which set off a healing response. There is an increase in cellular immunity, IL-2 production, NK cell activity, and macrophage phagocytosis. It can modulate cortisol and other hormones.

- The special point Pee Gun can be used for all masses; it is located 3 ½ cun lateral to the inferior tip of the spinous process of the twelfth thoracic vertebra. Burn 14 X red bean size moxa every 7 days, on the side of the body affected by cancer. A *cun* is an "inch" - but the actual length varies from patient to patient and from one area on the body to another - it is proportional to various anatomical parts in the region. For example on the face it is the width of the eye, but on the scalp it is $1/12^{th}$ the distance from the front hairline to the back hairline. Moxa is made from the leaf of the mugwort plant *Artemesia vulgaris*, and when lit it slowly smolders, warming the acupuncture point. Moxibustion is an alternative to needling or can be used with needles. While its smoke is relatively non-toxic, I usually would rather needle the point and then put an infrared heat lamp over the area to warm the needles gently, which has the same effect of increasing the Yang and dispersing the stagnant qi.

- Turtle technique on a mass involves needles from 3 directions towards the center, and ginger moxibustion to a fourth needle into the center of a tumor. The moxa is burned in little cones set on a thin slice of fresh ginger root, which has several holes punched through it with a toothpick; this is even more Yang than plain moxa.

- Primary points to consider, in the context of 8 Principles or 5 Element balancing would include PC-6 and HT-7, GV 12 and 13 coupled with BL-38.

- Secondary points which activate chi and blood with LI-4 and LV-3 (the Four Gates) plus ST-36, SP-6, GV-4 and 6, CV-4 & 6, LU-9, LV-2.

- Stimulate the Yang to invigorate the chi and dissolve stagnant blood with the master and coupled points of the Du channel SI-3 and BL-62, and consider also GV-4, 14, 20 & 26, BL-23 and GB-20. Needle and moxa BL-17 and 43 and GV-9 and14 to strengthen a Yang deficient patient.

- Prosperity treatment uses 4 points 1 cun above, below and lateral to the umbilicus. Insert and turn clockwise starting from CV 7 for constipation. Insert and turn counter-clockwise starting with ST 25 Left for diarrhea. Supplemental constipation points include GB-34 & ST-36.

- For vomiting consider CV-12 & 22, ST-12, PC-6, ST-36 and HT-1.

- To support the bone marrow use the Sea of Marrow points GV-15, 16, 19 & 20. Other anemia points to needle are BL-14 & 17 & 20, GV-4 & 14, CV-4 & 12, LV-13, SP-8 & 10, LI-11; moxibustion may be used on ST 36, SP-6 & 10, CV-4 and GV-4. For blood deficiency use Chong Mo master and control points PC-6 with contralateral SP-4.

- Ascites can be moderated with ST-22 and CV-9

- Acute leukemia treatment - BL-18 & 23, GB-39.

QI GONG

Qi gong is a traditional Chinese practice cultivating a balance of yi -intention or consciousness, with qi - vital energy - to balance mind and body. Qi gong exercises are thought to move energy through the organs, and qi gong masters are said to be able to move the energy in patients by the force of their own will. I have seen demonstrations of qi gong which are very dramatic. I have experienced the movement of palpable energy from a distance by a qi gong master. Chinese research points to improved immune function - macrophage phagocytosis, white blood cell counts, CD-20, IL-2 and NK cell activity. Cancer patients undergoing self-control qi gong therapy also demonstrated decreased inflammation, improved appetite, regularized bowel function, normalized liver function, increased self-healing, and weight gain. Late-stage cancer patients gain increased survival time. It is interesting that qi gong training is said to return the person to their "original self", releasing them from their "socialized self". This mirrors the concept of reinforcing the inner direction of psychic enegy versus the outward directed energy, which is a focus of the psychotherapeutic approach of LeShan and Simenton. The chi energy of qi gong healing is the same universal healing energy used in Reiki and Healing Touch.

HOMEOPATHY

Homeopathy is a 200 year old system of using very dilute substances to provoke the healing systems of the body to higher function. Vaccination is a crude form of homeopathy, using a tiny dose of a specially processed substance that in a full dose of the active substance would have provoked the actual disease in a healthy patient. It is 'like-cures-like', using a triggering dose to get the body to work on the problem by giving it a dose of information about the disease.

It is very gentle, and results can be very gratifying. It is highly individualized, and a good homeopathic prescription takes some time and thought by an experienced practitioner.

- In all cases consider *Scirrhus* 30 - 200 CH or *Carcinosum* 30 - 200 CH weekly. This does not mean give it slavishly to every patient though!

- For cachexia consider *Arsenicum iodatum* 3X after food.

- Other leading remedies are *Euphorbium* for pain, *Arsenicum album* for drug toxicity and in palliation, *Hydrastis canadensis* for constipation and lethargy, *Conium maculatum* for hard masses.

- Dr. Robin Murphy, N.D. has written an excellent alphabetical repertory with a good section on cancer under "Generals".

- Dr. Ivo Bianchi, M.D. uses Heel brand "homotoxicology" products such as *Gallium-Heel* 20 drops morning and night for 2 months, to be repeated 3 to 4 times a year, for prevention - to halt oncogenesis, in cancer therapy, and to promote detoxification; Lymphomyosot for lymphatic drainage; *Glyoxal-compositum* to neutralize toxins released by damaged cellular processes - do not repeat too often, allow time for it to work; *Traumeel* to ease pain and speed healing of mucositis induced by chemotherapy.

There are many self-help books available, and progressive pharmacies are once again carrying over-the-counter homeopathic remedies. Homeopathic physicians such as naturopathic doctors are essential for best results in treating serious illness, and for advice on combining homeopathic products with other medicines.

PSYCHOLOGY

Every experienced physician knows that a lot of patients in their practice are expressing physical illness related to psychological and emotional factors. These are apects of the mind, which is seated in the brain. Everybody has complex thoughts and feelings based on prior learning, imagination, hormonal balance, nutritional status and culture.

Grieving starts the moment the patient hears the word "cancer" from their doctor. People tend to go into denial, then anger, bargaining, depression and helplessness, before they can emerge with some resolution. It is normal to fear death, loss of control, pain, weakness, medicalization of one's life, social ostracism, financial loss, and so on. It is important to address these concerns, give stress-busting techniques to relieve anxiety, and clarify a person's self-image.

Dying tends to obscure the fact they still have living to do. All living persons should be working towards emotional and mental health, through self-effort and professional therapy. Personally, I like neuro-linguistic (NLP) psychology and Time-Line therapy, forms of cognitive therapy proven to relieve clinical anxiety. Good psychotherapy opens up a person to new expression of their physical, psychological and spiritual selves.

The rational and scientific evaluation of psychosocial interventions in cancer is in its infancy. Clearly measures which will be useful will have to have potent *psychogenicity*, the ability to stimulate lasting and major change in the thoughts, moods, habits and lifestyle of these cases. The response to the threat of cancer should be a realization of a need for significant change, a willingness to act, an application to self-help strategies, and achievement of quality experiences in the new modes of being.

- Carl O. Simenton and others have shown there is real survival value in positive affirmations, meditation, creative visualization, peer support, professional psychological facilitation, and therapy. Other de-stressing techniques may include yogic belly breathing, skin temperature biofeedback, and autogenic progressive relaxation.

- Feelings of loneliness, worthlessness, and fear are common inner conflicts. Increasing self-worth attitudes can improve self-caring and create an indomitable will to live. Poor outcomes are associated with a helplessness or hopelessness response to the cancer diagnosis and treatment plan. Unmitigated stress flattens the daily diurnal peaks of the adrenal stress hormone cortisol.

- LeShan, Booth, Thomas and others have described a cancer personality profile. There is a tendency to value and live through others, with most thoughts and activities being outwardly directed. "Type C" behaviour pattern is associated with higher risk of developing cancer, and a less favorable course of the disease. Patients with this coping style rarely express anger, anxiety, fear or sadness. They are unassertive, appeasing, yielding and very cooperative. They tend to be overly concerned with meeting the needs of others, and do not put their own needs forward.

- People who embrace and feel good about their cancer therapy tend to have far less side-effects than those who fear it and have morbid expectations. Anxiety and depression set a patient up for a poorer response and more harm from chemotherapy.

- Pain is much more easily borne by a patient who feels hopeful in facing a challenge than one whose thoughts dwell on what is lost and what is threatened by their disease. Hope is not something to avoid arousing, it is essential, for the physical therapeutic value as well as for psychological well-being.

- A weekly support group and self-hypnosis for pain was associated with doubling of life-span in advanced stage IV breast cancer, ovarian cancer and melanoma. This work by Spiegel from 1989 has not been confirmed in subsequent studies, but certainly quality of life improves, if survival does not.

- Particularly vulnerable are patients who lack a significant social support network. Patients who report a poor level of social well-being show higher pre-surgical levels of the angiogenesis cytokine VEGF.

- Cancer patients need to learn how to live fully - as LeShan says "love, laugh, play, learn, sing praises and exercise".
  To be filled with joy, gratitude and love is to be healed, whatever the circumstances of the physical body.

- Love is all there is. Love is the only true meaning in life and death. The old term "placebo response" is now being called a "meaning response". People heal when they find meaning in their life. When they express their inner selves, they can remember love, speak their truth, and move into a still and sacred place where they co-create a reality where they are kind to themselves and all others.

SPIRITUALITY

Because it is a life-and-death struggle to overcome cancer, it is a spiritual process. Treating this "ghost in the machine" is not an area of expertise of most medical practitioners.

I do not believe there can be "false hope". I believe despair and fear to be false emotions. Remember *fear is faith in evil*. Place your faith in something positive. Hope is life-enhancing on a daily level, and many people also have hope concerning a possible eternity.

A diagnosis of an incurable disease can create false hopelessness.
A patient does not have to accept pain, abandonment, suffering or giving up being productive only because the future is uncertain.

- Stress is lessened by reasserting personal control . Doing "everything that can be done" just feels better than giving up.
  A reminder of our mortality can bring profound meaning back into the lives of patients and their families.

- A terminal diagnosis means a person has time to prepare for their death. Resolution of conflicts and the giving and receiving of forgiveness are possible gifts.

- Expressive therapies such as music or art help modulate neuro-endocrine-immune parameters.

- Religious faith, prayers, rituals and spiritual practices are coping mechanisms positively associated with better outcomes. People who have faith in a higher power, and particularly those who attend church or practice their religion actively have measurably lower rates of complications, less need for medications, and tend to survive longer with more quality of life. People of faith tend to feel peace, assurance, meaning and well-being which allows them to embrace life. Faith in an afterlife or spiritual survival does correlate with an increased fighting spirit seen in cancer survivors. They fear death less, yet fight to survive more.

- Simple mind-body techniques may include compassionate heart-focussed meditation, journaling, or breathing exercises.

OXYGEN THERAPIES

- Ozone (O3) is a highly reactive form of oxygen which may be insufflated into the rectum or bubbled through 50 to 100 ml of blood which is then returned to the body (autohemotherapy). It up-regulates the immune system if given in low doses, increases superoxide dismutase (SOD), increases catalase, and detoxifies the liver. Ozone is radiosensitizing.

- Hydrogen peroxide (H2O2) is used orally, or intravenously at 0.03%, and has significant risks. Hydrogen peroxide, even that produced by our own macrophage immune cells, permanently inactivates our NK immune cells - which we need to kill cancer cells. Dark field microscopy suggests peroxide may trigger very dangerous changes in the blood. I do not recommend H2O2.

- Hyperbaric oxygen therapy (HBO2T) is breathing of 100% oxygen at elevated pressure to super-saturate the body with oxygen, and force it deep into cells. Tumors do use fermentation to make energy without oxygen, but also burn fats and carbohydrates with oxygen. They are NOT poisoned by oxygen as some people suggest. Some have also suggested HBO2T would increase tumor growth due to its power to stimulate increased angiogenesis. HBO2T has no net benefit in treating cancer, but may safely be given if needed for other medical reasons. HBO2T must never be used within 4 weeks of radiation therapy.

DMSO

Di-methyl sulfoxide is a powerful solvent with analgesic, vulnerary (wound healing) and anti-inflammatory properties. It is useful also as a carrier to move medications through cell membranes. Intravenous use is more risky than orally or by enema. It can cause halitosis or bad breath – in this case a garlic oyster smell and taste, headache, dizziness, nausea and sedation. It may be a useful adjunct in leukemia, uterine and cervical cancers. Methyl sulfonyl methane (MSM) in capsule form may provide many similar benefits, and may be better in bladder cancer. MSM is great for arthritic pain, hay fever, strengthens hair and nails, and has many other beneficial side-effects.

EDTA CHELATION

Chelation is an intravenous treatment which removes toxic heavy metals such as lead. EDTA chelation has been used, amid some controversy, for cardiovascular disease. Unanticipated benefits in cancer status have been reported. Chelation may inhibit free radicals and enhance immune defenses. It is safe when administered by a physician certified by the American College for the Advancement of Medicine (ACAM). Take it 1 to 3 times per week, supplement vitamin C, B complex, zinc, selenium, and anything else the routine blood analyses indicate to be imbalanced.

714X

Gaston Naessens argues that this chemical source of nitrogen for the body will stop the cancer cells from producing "co-carcinogenic K factor" (CKF) which protects them from immune cells. It contains camphor, organic salts, ethanol and water. 714X is injected into the lymph nodes for 3 series of 21 days each, spaced by three days off, then boosters as needed. Do not combine with vitamin E or vitamin B12 supplementation, which decrease its effectiveness. It is also incompatible with anti-angiogenics.

SHORT-WAVE DIATHERMY

Dr. John Bastyr, ND said that passing 13 meter short-wave radiation through a tumor will dissolve it. The patient needs to be fit to handle the toxic debris from rapid tumor lysis (break-up). Consider also diathermy to the pituitary gland.

RIFE RAY

Royal Rife in San Diego in 1934 demonstrated an electromagnetic therapy termed the Rife Ray which could be tuned to specific frequencies to destroy specific disease organisms, including viruses, within living tissue. Rife build a uniqely powerful light microscope and observed a viral size organism he associated with cancer cells, and observed his ray killing them. He then treated human tumors, with claimed success, but was stopped by the American Medical Association by 1939.
Some of my patients and colleagues have Rife devices, but I am unable to confirm their efficacy. I do not believe they cause any harm.

HYPERTHERMIA

Cells with a low pH (high in acid) or with nutritional deficiencies, such as hypoxic tumor cells, are more sensitive to heat damage than healthy cells. Rapidly proliferating cells are also slower to develop a tolerance to heat over 42°C. Cancer cells are deficient in "chaperone proteins" including heat shock proteins (HSP). HSP cover the hydrophobic portions of amino acid chains emerging from the cell's endoplasmic reticulum, and later assist new proteins to achieving the proper tertiary structure (shape). Heat induces apoptosis via intracellular triggers and branched chain polysaccharide alterations, and can also induce necrosis. Core body temperature elevation may be safely tolerated to about 42 to 42.5 degrees Celsius. Core body hyperthermia is not recommended in cases of liver injury or disease. Destruction of malignant tissue is expected in the range of 42 to 44°C. For each degree above 41°C half the amount of time is needed to kill the same number of cells. At 44° a malignant tumor may be destroyed in about 30 minutes. Dr. George Crile Jr. of Cleveland estimates cancerous cells are destroyed at temperatures about 3°C lower than that which will destroy adjacent normal tissue, at any given duration of exposure.

Hyperthermia in the range of 41 to 42°C for 30 to 40 minutes, or 2°C. above their baseline for 30 to 60 minutes, produces an anti-neoplastic immune response. There is up-regulation of NK cell activity and mitogenesis, increased interleukins IL-1 and IL-2, increased circulating CD4/CD8 cell ratios, and increased circulating peripheral mononuclear cells. Diaphoresis is also detoxifying. Hyperthermia is radio-sensitizing, by inhibition of repair of chromosome aberrations and single strand DNA breaks, which results in apoptosis of radiation injured cells.In 1891 Dr. William Coley began injecting a mixture of streptococcal bacteria endotoxins into 140 patients with advanced sarcomas to induce an artificial fever. His "metabolic hyperthermia" had positive responses directly related to the temperature reached and the duration of the fever. Dr. Issels carried on the practice with bacterial lysates. At the turn of the 20th Century Dr. Westermark developed whole body hyperthermia in hot baths. Others worked with short wave diathermy, microwave, infrared and ultrasound heating. In 1976 Dr. Leon Parks, a cardiothoracic surgeon introduced hyperthermia by extracorporeal circulation using computerized perfusion technology. This method results in pain palliation and effective reversal of tumor growth in a significant number of patients. One of my esteemed colleagues, Dr. Garrett Swetlikoff, ND, who for many years was my personal physician, uses hyperthermia in his practice. The Heckel HT2000 whole body hyperthermia unit uses infrared A and a thermal insulation blanket to reach a core body temperature over 43 degrees Centigrade in sessions of 1 to 2 hours.

ELECTRICAL THERAPY

A small electrical current applied to a tumor has an antineoplastic effect, by normalizing cell proliferation rates. Cancer cells tend to have an abnormally low trans-membrane potential (TMP) which will increase with direct current (DC) application of less than 10 volts. Cancer cells have a low voltage of about 15 - 20 millivolts. Normal cells average 75 - 90 millivolts. Normal non-dividing cells will respond to DC with a lowering of their TMP.

The effect is greatest when the anode electrode is applied to the tumor. Acid and chlorine forms at the anode, alkali plus hydrogen forms at the cathode, and the cancer in the middle depolarizes, then dies.

The optimum current is 7.5 volts DC, 20 milliamperes, to a level of 35 -100 coulombs per cubic centimeter of tumor. Pads may be applied to superficial tumors for percutaneous stimulation, or electrodes can be applied to acupuncture needles for deeper tumors. Stimulation is applied for 15 to 30 minutes. Large tumors may take 100 milliamperes of current for up to 4 hours, for a dose of up to 100 coulombs of electrical energy. The treatment stings, so local anesthetic medication may be used.

The ideal tumor for this therapy is superficial and under 5 cm. in diameter. The lysis products provoke a favorable immune response. The fragments are ideal for processing by the macrophage immune cells.

The short-term response rate may be 85%. Long-term survival is higher with this adjunctive therapy in lung, esophageal liver and kidney cancers. In China this treatment is used in hundreds of hospitals, with galvanic current applied to platinum electrodes inserted into the tumor under ultrasound guidance. Incisions may be made under local anaesthetic. In Europe this has been pioneered by Nobel laureate Professor Bjorn Nordenstrom of Sweden and Dr. Rudolf Pekar of Austria. Dr. Pekar claims a 3 year remission rate of 73%. Chinese reports indicate about 35% complete remissions, 43% partial remissions, 15% unchanged, and only 7% experiencing progression of their disease. The Chinese say they see about 70% 3 year survival in total, for a wide variety of cancers.

After galvanotherapy the tumor cells may be seen to re-differentiate into fibroblasts and repair the area.

Electrotherapy has little effect in advanced disease with metastases, and does not inhibit the tendency to metastasize.

THE DIBELLA PROTOCOL

Recently this elderly Italian physiologist presented a protocol for evaluation, based on anecdotal evidence of good results. It combines melatonin with bromocriptine and somatostatin (or its synthetic analogue octrotide). Patients loved it, but the scientists did not. Perhaps this is yet another case of a healer who thought his medicine was the cure, when it was his own personality and art as a physician at work.

ANTINEOPLASTINS

Dr. Stanislaw Burzynski, MD, PhD developed two synthetic peptide (amino acid chain) formulations he named 'antineoplastins', which switch off oncogenes and switch on tumor suppressor genes. He found these naturally occurring peptides and organic acids tend to be low in the urine of cancer patients. They are not toxic. The average dose of A10 fraction is 7.7 g/kg/day, and the As2-1 fraction is given at 0.36 g/kg/day. After 20 years of harrassment by the USA Food and Drug Administration (FDA), he is now conducting approved trials through his Houston, Texas clinic. He appears to have the most success with brain and prostate cancers.

MAGNETICS

Magnets of 650 gauss static field strength may be used for 1 to 2 hours daily. Magnetic therapy dates back to the discovery of natural magnets in the earth in ancient China, balls of crude iron called 'lode stones'. The Chinese were the first to discover the magnetic compass, using a sliver of magnetized iron. The earth has a strong magnetic field, and every cell and most large molecules in them has some electrical charge which tends to want to line up with the magnetic field. When we live in artificial environments with electrical wires and concrete with iron rebar grids, and so on, we are blocked from our natural magnetic field, and may have strong and disorganized fields all around us. It is recommended that we not have electrical appliances such as clock radios near our heads when we sleep.

Nikken of Japan is the world leader in medical and health magnetic products, to wear, sleep on, and use therapeutically. They make the *Pi-Mag* water treatment system which makes water thinner, by breaking down the clumping of water into smaller 'micro-clusters'. This water is a super solvent for better detoxification. A similar concept is used in magnetic laundry discs which can be used instead of soap in a clothes or dishwasher – the water is able to penetrate better, like a dry-cleaning solvent, but without the chemicals. Magnets relieve pain, improve sleep and speed healing processes.

UKRAIN

Ukrain or NSC-631570 is a semi-synthetic compound of thiophosphoric acid triaziridide and an alkaloid chelidonine from the traditional liver herb *Chelidonium majus*. It has been used for about 20 years in Austria. The National Cancer Institute in the USA has found it active against many cancer cell types, including adenocarcinomas, epithelial carcinomas, sarcomas, melanoma and lymphomas.

Ukrain selectively accumulates in tumor cells, where it is directly cytolytic and cytostatic, inhibits topoisomerases I and II, inhibits synthesis of DNA, RNA and proteins. Ukrain induces apoptosis by activation of endodesoxyribonucleases. Ukrain initially increases oxygen consumption in cells, but later it returns to normal in healthy cells but stops completely in the cancer cells!

Ukrain in small doses is a biological response modifier (BRM) which means it is immune-stimulating. It can activate NK cells, improve the CD4/CD8 ratios, and increase phagocytosis by white blood cells.

The dose is commonly 5 to 20mg daily to weekly, intravenously or intramuscularly, usually 2 or 3 times a week. It is best to avoid mixing it directly with other products, and to inject each 5 ml x 5 mg ampoule slowly over a minute or more. A common strategy is to use 5 mg once a week as a BMR, alternating with 20 mg later in the week for a cancer cytolytic effect. Do not mix with cortisone, digitalis, sulphonamide antibiotics or sulfonyl urea antidiabetic drugs.

Ukrain is well-tolerated, with only moderate toxicity. There is no cumulative toxicity or late effects. Allergic or anaphylactic reactions are not seen. Ukrain is not recommended in pregnancy, breastfeeding, in growing children, or during high fever. Tumor markers may fluctuate early in therapy. Tumors may swell reversibly early in therapy, so be cautious with cancers within the skull.

Ukrain may cause some nausea, tumor swelling, dizziness, depression, insomnia, drowsiness, fatigue, apathy, restlessness, sweats, shivering, itching, increased urination, stabbing pains, tingling sensations, burning feeling in the tumor, and tumor hardening. These are due to tumor lysis releasing toxic matter, and will disappear as the tumor is removed.

Consider Ukrain in cancer of the breast, pancreas, colon, bladder, prostate, ovary, cervix, endometrium (uterus), lung, testes, head and neck, lymphoma and melanoma.
Phase II studies show a doubling of median survival time in advanced pancreatic cancer, used alone or with chemotherapy.

IMMUNE THERAPIES

Cancer cells form all the time, and the immune system removes them safely almost all of the time. There is always some element of immune failure when cancer becomes a disease.

Immune therapies are limited by the fact that most cancer cells are able to disguise their abnormality until they are very well established. Clearly most common epithelial cancers - carcinomas - show a very late immune response, and often their mutation rate exceeds the plasticity of the immune system to adapt. Without immune modifiers, the immune system hasn't a chance of picking up on the abnormalities until the patient is very sick. The cancer gets a big lead off, and the immune system can rarely catch up in time to prevent severe damage or death.

Recall from Chapter One that a huge volume of the DNA genetic code in every cell is made up of virus information, virus promoter sequences, and cancer-provoking oncogenes and proto-oncogenes. When cancer gets mature, and highly mutated, the viral overload can express and be the final step which destroys life.

Any inflammation, infection, parasite or other immune stressor can tip the balance in a very ill cancer patient. There are many cancer fighting immune therapies that have been used, and more in active development. This is potentially the most promising new direction for contemporary cancer research. Until we can get reliable and specific anti-cancer vaccines, the general immune status of our cancer patients remains a central concern for naturopathic physicians.

The modern level of cleanliness, and the use of vaccinations and immunizations to avoid childhood and infectious diseases has been linked to the modern epidemics of immmune disorders. Kids who are exposed to more germs and dirt have less allergies, less asthma, and so on. It is possible our drive to have a safe and sterile environment is making our immune systems weak, and contributing to our inability to deal with cancer cells as they form. We need an active reticulo-endothelial system, hardened by exposure to infections, to create immunity to the next disease we encounter.

Natural immunity can be raised by using cross-reacting antigens. The first immunization success was the introduction of cowpox inoculation to make antibodies effective against smallpox. Jenner introduced this in 1796, and in 180 years smallpox was extinct. This is the very principle on which the great medical art and science of homeopathy is based - the use of "Similars" to provoke the body to heal itself.

Immune treatments may modulate or supplement interleukins, cytokines, and viral-blocking interferons.

BCG immunization is a non-specific immune enhancer from a form of tuberculosis bacteria common in cattle. A suspension of 75 mg live bacillus per ml. is smeared into a 5 cm square of 20 skin scratches every four days for a month, then once weekly, for courses of ten to sixteen applications. BCG may also be injected into tumors such as melanoma at doses of 0.05 to 0.20 ml of the suspension per nodules.

Coley's toxins from the bacteria *Streptococcus pyogenes* and *Serratia marcescens*; preparations from *Corynebacterium parvum* or *Corynebacterium pseudodipthericum*; staphage lysates from *Staphylococcus aureus* or *Staphylococcus epidermidis*; vaccines from *Eschericia coli, Klebsiella pneumoniae, Haemophilus influenzae, Moraxella catarrhalis, Streptococcus pneumoniae, Streptococcus salivarius, & Streptococcus pyogenes* induce a cytokine APO-2 ligand, which is like tumor necrosis factor (TNF) but even more active in killing cancer cells. Also used are DNCB extract or MBVmixed bacterial vaccine. *Corynebacterium parvum* bacteria preparation is superior to BCG for stimulating macrophages. It is given intravenously, intra-tumor, or subcutaneous by two to four injections in the lymphatic drainage field around tumors, totalling 2 mg for the first treatment, then at 2 to 4 mg per treatment. For fever, hydrothorax, cor pulmonale, thrombocytopenia, liver disorder or severe weakness consider raising the dose up to 8 mg.

The Polish *Polyvaccinum preparation*, or the simpler and cheaper *Respivax* mixed respiratory vaccine have long been used by doctors in British Columbia, and have induced remissions in advanced cancer cases. A typical protocol would be 0.05 to 0.75 cc of vaccine injected subcutaneously, sufficient to evoke a red flare (erythema) up to 5 cm. in diameter within 24 hours. A good response is often accompanied by a mild fever.

MTH-68/N - a promising immune response modifier using paramyxovirus from chickens, weakened and modified, and given by a nasal spray. This attenuated *Newcastle disease* virus is harmless to humans, only occasionally provoking a "pink-eye" sort of conjunctivitis. Advanced cancer patients frequently experience disease stabilization, reduction in pain, improved performance status, and sometimes get full remissions after several months. Developed and used in Budapest, Hungary by Laszlo and Eva Csatary.

Any viral vaccine can provoke increased non-specific immunity. An example is the common MRV - mixed respiratory virus vaccine.

Naturopathic physicians for generations have used immune gland extracts of animal origin. Thymus gland has been given as capsules or by injection to activate or modulate T-cells. Thymosin 8 mg may be injected every two to three days for one to two months, including during chemo or radiation therapies. If thymic factor is substituted, the dose is about 30 mg. Polyerga is a pig spleen peptide extract which at 300 to 500 mg daily can increase white blood cells and their output of gamma interferon. This inhibits metastasis, improves appetite, reduces pain, improves overall vitality, and increases survival time.

Remember surgery is very immunosuppressive, as are many chemotherapy drugs.

Isopathic preparations have often been made from the patient's own blood, urine or tissue. Tumor biopsy tissue must first be inactivated. Tissue is pulverized into a suspension and is injected in the deltoid muscle on the upper arm at doses of 0.2 to 0.3 ml. every five to seven days for five to seven treatments. This may be repeated after two to four months.

Liver flukes are not "The Cause of All Cancers" as Hulda Clarke claims, but they are associated with cholangio-carcinoma in the bile ducts. Parasites in general are very common, and while the healthy patient need not fear about a few critters in the bowels, a very ill patient may benefit from removing an infestation that is robbing them of nutrition.

Histamine via H2 receptors mediates natural killer cell anticancer activity. Histamine blocks macrophage and monocyte respiratory burst of hydrogen peroxide and other ROS compounds which would otherwise irreversibly inhibit NK cell cytotoxicity and induce apoptosis in NK cells. Histamine has been shown to synergize with IL-2 and IFNa in treatment of melanoma and leukemia.

The strength of the immune system can be degraded by stress, whether physical, psychological and emotional. The immune cells have receptors on their surface and respond to neurotransmitters, the chemicals of thought and mood. This relatively new field of study is called psychoneuroimmunology. In the 1920's the nutrition genius Francis Pottinger studied the nutriton and health of many Stone Age hunter -gatherer remnant societies from Africa to the Arctic. He proposed a theory that immune system cancers such as leukemia, lymphoma and multiple myeloma arose in persons who are parasympathetic dominant. The Autonomic nervous system has 2 parts, the Sympathetic which turns on the stress arousal reaction of "fight or flight", and the Parasympathetic which turns it off.

Lymphocytes in the spleen and thymus gland have receptors for parasympathetic neurotransmitters. These people tend to be somewhat lethargic or laid back types, susceptible to viruses, and overreactive to infections and inflammation triggers.

Conversely, Pottinger thought solid tumors occurred with sympathetic dominance, that is in people who are highly stressed, with low immune reactivity and low digestive function, including low pancreatic enzymes.

Determining the relative dominance of these two arms of this primitive and subconscious part of our nervous system may give a new strategy to heal the whole person. Acupuncture is one method to rapidly balance these two arms of the autonomic nervous system.

The Krebiozen therapy espoused by Professor Andrew C. Ivy was never properly tested, and remains the most interesting innovation in cancer immunology history. Made by injecting horses with the *Actinomyces* fungus from a non-cancerous tumor in cattle called "lumpy-jaw", the resulting serum yielded an "anti-growth hormone" and would stimulate reticuloendothelial immunity in human cancer patients. Modern naturopathic physicians and homeopaths using Sanum pleomorphic remedies from *Actinomyces* should find this a clue for further research.

Dr. Enderlein has professed that small microbes living in the blood can assemble into this Actinomycetes fungus in the metabolic ruin of advanced systemic cancer.

Gruner, Glover, Hatsumi, Issels and others have identified a filterable creature in human blood they call a cancer virus, or a bacterium of the size of a virus.

Virginia Livingstone in California makes a vaccine against an organism she calls *Progenitor crytocides* which she feels is a cause of cancer.

Enderlein, Gaston Naessens, Royal Rife, and others show us them in human blood under dark field microscopes fitted with proper condensors. Pleomorphic commensal organisms living inside us which can spontaneously generate disease germs in our blood - this is very unsettling to those who try to make a Universal Law out of the Germ Theory of Louis Pasteur. Pasteur recognized the *milieu* was "everything" Do we not have the "germs" of disease in every cell in the form of virus DNA fused right into our own chromosomes? Is it possible this mass of viral material, including oncogenes, in our DNA might "sponateously generate" germs under conditions seen in an advanced malignant tumor? I believe immunosuppression might trigger superinfections, inflammation and ultimately cause cancer to flourish.

The pleomorphic theories of Gaston Naessens and Professor Enderlein suggest we carry pre-viral elements in our cells, which can assemble into viruses and fungi from within our bodies, when we are toxic and metabolically disordered. If Enderlein is correct, there may also be fungal pathogens latent in the blood or deeper inside the cells.

We do not merely give antifungal and antiviral medication - we work on the biochemical *terrain*, the nutritional and physical environment of the cells. Naturopathic immune therapies rebalance the entire ecology to regulate inflammation, enhance immune cell surveillance for cancer cells, and control bacteria, parasites, and viruses.

Naturopathic approaches to immune support include thymus products, mushroom polysaccharides, chloryphyll, plant sterols and sterolins, and psychoneuroimmunology.

Vitamin A derivative retinoic acid will decrease viral DNA such as the human papilloma virus (HPV) inside cells.

Homeopathics such as *Thymuline and Engystol* are excellent for viral control. I use them in cancer, but also to prevent or treat influenza and other viral illness. The Sanum homeopathic remedies based on Enderlein's fungal pathology concepts are remarkably strong and effective medicines.

Remember that immune tonics work best when given early in the day, such as one dose at breakfast and another before lunch.

MISCELLANEOUS

There are an infinity of weird and wacky cancer "cures" of uncertain benefit. I have no direct experience or knowledge to recommend trying or referring patients for these approaches, some of which may be valuable - but I cannot say which. Please get advice from a practitioner experienced with a therapy before trusting your life to it:

- Cesium salts to alter cellular acidity
- Bestatin UBX from Streptomyces olivereticuli
- Live cell therapy with fetal cells or stem cells.
- Thymus glandular injections
- Amino acids such as Jinlong capsules
- Laetrile, also known as amygdalin, sarcarcinase, nitriloside or Vitamin B17
- Insulin shock therapy
- Wobenzyme N - pancreatin , bromelain and rutin
- Radiofrequency tumor ablation, including the Rife machine.
- Electrotherapy such as the Beck Zapper device
- MGN-3 with shiitake enzymes and modified arabinoxylan.
- Macrobiotic diet

A few which I really doubt have any merit:
- Morinda citrifolia or Noni juice.
- Sun Soup a patented herbal food with shiitake.
- Hulda Clark's parasite treatment
- Chondriana crystals
- Colostrum transfer factors
- Immuno-Augmentative Therapy (IAT)
- Germanium sesquioxide supplementation

"The universe is full of magical things patiently waiting for our wits to grow sharper."
the essayist Eden Phillpotts

Chapter Eight -   COMPLICATIONS & EMERGENCIES

The management of advanced cancers requires vigilance for morbidity which can rapidly turn to mortality. Cancer patients die prematurely of hemorrhage, obstructions, infection, malnutrition and organ failures. Pathological fractures, ascites, bleeding and seizures can be the first sign of advanced disease. Skilled naturopathic physicians can treat some of these issues, and be alert to refer others for definitive medical care.

PAIN

The best defense against pain is to control and remove the cancer! Detoxification is also very appropriate, if gently scaled to the vitality of the patient. Natural anti-inflammatories that are as effective as synthetic drugs, and safer, are easily obtained. Anti-inflammatory drugs can reduce the need for dose–escalation of opioids such as morphine, preventing the constipation and stupor those heavy drugs bring. Reducing inflammation has the beneficial side-effect of slowing tumor growth.

True analgesics of great strength are not so readily found in the natural pharmacy. Much has been written about the need for humane and aggressive use of drug cocktails with controversial addictive drugs such as heroin in end-stage disease. Certainly we need to do all we can to ease suffering, and fear of drug addiction is not a sensible reason to refuse opiates for a person in their last days.

I have often been able to help people die in comfort with no drugs whatsoever. Fortunately the mind is sometimes mightier than matter.

- Assess pain on a scale from 1 to 10, or with kids use a visual scale such as happy vs. sad faces.   Ask if the pain level is "acceptable".

- Acupuncture is very helpful for moderate cancer pain. Acupuncture is best when prescribed within the context of authentic TCM. Commonly used pain-releiving points are LI-4, BL-60, ST-36, SP-4, GB-20, GB-43, PC-6 and LV-3. Think of KI-7 for bone pain. TENS, massage, injections and heat can be more effective if applied to nerves at acupuncture points.

- Detoxification releives pain - detox with raw food, fresh juices and liver tonifying herbs such as burdock, dandelion root, milk thistle, Xiao Chai Hu Tang, or *Herbotox.*

- Coffee enemas are actually helpful for pain in a toxic cancer patient. Coffee enemas were listed in the Merck Manual until 1977, for a variety of conditions. About 4 to 6 ounces of cooled fresh-brewed coffee are placed in the rectal canal and retained. Caffeine and other constituents move up the hemorrhoidal veins to the portal vein and on into the liver, increasing the bile outflow. Overuse can cause deficiencies of vitamins A and E, loss of the electrolyte mineral sodium, and dehydration.

- Boswellic acid from frankincense gum *Boswellia serrata* or *B. carteri* is a powerful anti-inflammatory plant extract. It has also been shown to induce differentiation, induce apoptosis, and inhibit tumor cells. *Phytoprofen* from Thorne Research is a potent professional product using boswellic acid and other plants extracts for pain and inflammation.

- Cox-2 cycloxygenase inhibitors - such as cold-water fish omega 3 fatty acids, feverfew *Tanacetum parthenium*, scute *Scutellaria baicalensis*, rosemary, propolis, curcumin, and grapeseed proanthocyanins - help in reducing doses of narcotics, relieving side-effects of constipation, drowsiness, stupor, confusion.

- *Una de Gato* or cat's claw herb is used to reduce cancer pain, detoxifies, and boosts immune function too.

- *Panax pseudoginseng* or notoginseng relieves pain by moving 'stagnant blood'.

- Art therapy, relaxation techniques, counselling, prayer, psychotherapy, positive affirmations, visualization, guided imagery, and meditation are associated with reduced pain, improved sleep, and improved quality of life. Every effort should be made to encourage the patient to approach every life-threatening illness as a challenge which brings gifts and meaning. I often recommend reading *Love, Medicine & Miracles* by Bernie Siegel, MD

- Homeopathics *Euphorbium* or *Phosphoricum acidicum* 6 to 30 CH, every 2 hours. Secondary remedies: *Apis mellifica, Arsenicum album, Carcinosum, Colocynthis, Conium, Hydrastis.*

Tumors will crush organs, compress nerves, block up vessels and tubes and pressurize cavities. There is a time for high dose radiation about 400 rads per dose for 3 doses or for Prednisone (cortisone) steroids to shrink or "debulk" aggressive cancer.

LYMPHEDEMA - is a swelling caused by obstruction or loss of the lymphatic drainage. It is most common in an arm after mastectomy, surgery to remove a cancerous breast. However, lymph channels anywhere can be blocked by tumors, as well as by cutting or post-surgical and post-radiation scarring. Lymph is a fluid that leaks out of cells, percolates through tiny spaces, eventually being collected in small ducts, flowing through lymph nodes filled with immune cells monitoring the cellular debris floating by. Eventually it all flows into the thoracic duct in the chest to rejoin the bloodstream. Lymphedema is an accumulation of fluid and protein. This protein acts as a colloid or gel matrix, holding fluid by osmosis.

Lymphedema after mastectomy causes arm swelling, pain, immobility, and even small injuries can precipitate inflammation (lymphangitis) and infection (cellulitis).

A Juzo compression sleeve can help, as can pneumatic pumps or manual drainage massage. Registered massage therapists with advanced training in lymphology should be treating all cases.

Naturopathic physicians may utilize German complex homeopathics such as *Lymphmyosot* from Heel and botanical/homeopathics such as *Lymphdiaral* from Pascoe Pharmacie. Fresh *Ceanothus spp.* "red root" removes waste from the lymphatic system.

American trained naturopathic physicians use high dose protease (protein dissolving) and lipase (fat dissolving) enzymes from Tyler Encapsulations, on the advice of enzyme therapy luminary Dr. Howard Loomis.

TUMOR LYSIS SYNDROME - is a toxic overload of the kidneys due to aggressive treatment resulting in rapid necrosis. The metabolic load of rising potassium, phosphate, and uric acid and falling calcium results in acidosis and azotemia. Watch for cardiac arrythmias, arthritis, weakness, lethargy, tachypnea, or coma with deep Kussmaul respirations. Most commonly seen in acute leukemias and lymphomas. Monitor serum LDH enzyme as a marker of necrosis.

SUPERIOR VENA CAVA SYNDROME - is a compression of the vein returning blood from the head and thorax to the heart. Tumors in the mediastinum, next to the heart, are the culprit. These may include primary lymphomas or metastases to the mediastinal lymph nodes from lung or breast cancer. The earliest warning sign is facial edema, which can spread to the neck and upper extremities. Later cyanosis can appear, and there may be veinous distension visible on the chest.

PERICARDIAL TAMPONADE - is a fluid build-up in the pericardial sac to the point of limiting the filling of the heart in diastole with right-sided heart failure and diminished cardiac output. The patient will be anxious with oppressive chest discomfort, dyspnea, orthopnea, weakness, cough and dysphagia. There may be distended jugular veins with inspiratory swelling, faint heart sounds, tachycardia, weak arterial pulses, hypotension and pulsus paradox. There may be hepatomegaly and peripheral edema. A chest x-ray may show cardiomegaly with a "sac-like'"appearance, as well as pleural effusion.

INTRACRANIAL PRESSURE - may rise from brain and meningeal tumors to provoke symptoms such as headaches. Nausea and visual changes are also common, followed by personality changes, lethargy, and coma. Signs include papilledema, focal neurological deficits, seizures and possibly nuchal rigidity and pain. A dilated and fixed pupil indicates tentorial herniation, which will often progress to death by crushing the breathing centers in the brainstem.

SPINAL CORD CMPRESSION - can develop insidiously with muscle weakness, sensory disturbances, changes in bowel and bladder function, paresis. Paraplegia or quadriplegia can follow in as little as 12 to 24 hours.

ASCITES - may develop from portal hypertension caused by liver metastases as in colon or breast cancer, from peritoneal carcinomatosis as in ovarian, breast or GI adenoacarcinomas, and occassionally from malignant lymphomas in the abdomen. The patient may report swelling of the abdomen and/or dyspnea. Look for shifting abdominal dullness, and a palpable fluid wave. Therapeutic paracentesis (drainage of the fluid by needle with suction) can provoke severe protein deficits. We prescribe 5 servings of protein daily and monitor serum albumin.
Intraperitoneal instillation of radioactive P-32 can reduce ascites, provided there is no history of radiation to the area or major adhesions limiting the free flow of the fluids. Consider homeopathic *Apocyanum*.

ANEMIA - is common in many chronic diseases. We use iron citrate, folate, B12, and *Shiquan* to keep hemoglobin in the 11 - 12 range. Transfusions are needed if hemoglobin falls below 9 - 10, and allopaths may use erythropoeitin, a marrow stimulating hormone from the kidney (Procrit or Epigen) injected once weekly.

DISSEMINATED INTRAVASCULAR COAGULATION (DIC) - is a decline in fibrinogen and clotting factors leading to a hemmorhagic diathesis (bleeding). Neoplastic cells can release thromboplastin-like material, especially acute promyelocytic leukemia and prostate adenocarcinoma.

LEUKOSTASIS - is a syndrome where extreme levels of circulating leukemic blast cells, i.e. over 100,000/mm3, cause multiple infarcts and hemorrhages in the lungs and brain.

THROMBOCYTOPENIA - platelets below 20,000/mm3 from myelosuppression by radiotherapy or chemotherapy, from marrow replacement with tumor, or from intravascular coagulation. Lack of platelets to make a clot can lead to serious hemorrhages, often intracranial.

BLOOD CLOTS - cancers often make pro-coagulants such as cytokines, activators of clotting factors IX & X, increase platelet reactivity and cause venous stasis by local anatomical change. Prostate cancer is notorious for promoting blood clots, as are hormonal therapies such as Tamoxifen. Watch for petechiae, ecchymosis (bruising) and deep vein thrombosis. Natural control of coagulation may include gingko leaf *Gingko biloba*, fish oils, green tea, green leafy vegetables, horse chestnut *Aesculus hippocanastum*, red clover blossom *Trifolium repens* and compression stockings.

HEMORRHAGE - Tumors erode into blood vessels, angiogenesis can form weak and leaky vessels, necrotic areas can erode and bleed, and clotting can be severely disturbed by a variety of mechanisms. Yunnan Paiyao is an excellent treatment for a hemorrhagic diathesis. Consider also *Geranium maculatum* - spotted cranesbill and *Capsella bursa-pastoris* - sheperd's purse. Homeopathics such as *Phosphorus* can be added as adjuncts.

BOWEL OBSTRUCTION - may occur below the ileum with colorectal tumors, lymphomas, or peritoneal metastases from ovarian adenocarcinoma. Obstruction above the ileum may occur with esophageal, gastric, pancreatic, hepatocellular and biliary tumors. Watch for early satiety, cramping abdomenal pains, constipation and nausea. Vomiting may follow, becoming feculent. Signs include a distended tympanic abdomen, high-pitched and frequent bowel sounds. Later bowel sounds may be absent. Dehydration can occur from vomiting and from sequestration of fluid in the distended bowel loop – "third spacing".

CACHEXIA - is a metabolic rate increase mediated by cytokines and marked by increased glucose production, increased lipolysis and protein catabolism. Natural agents of great value include melatonin and EPA oils. Maintain adequate protein, calories, and exercise. Cachexia is not caused by poor appetite, but stimulating appetite with dilute hydrochloric acid (HCl), cannabis THC or vitamin B1 can be helpful.

HYPERCALCEMIA - can result from bone mets, vitamin D metabolites made by tumors, increased PGE2, dehydration, and very rarely from tumor production of parathyroid hormone releasing protein (PTH-RP). Symptoms may be weakness, fatigue, irritability, depression, nausea, vomiting, abdomenal pain and reversible coma.

BONE METASTASES - many cancers go into the bones - for example 70 to 80% of breast cancer mets and about 70% of prostate cancer mets. Gnawing pain, usually worse at night, may wake the person up from sleep. Pain may become sharp with weight-bearing, relieved by rest. Bone scans are the best method to screen for bony mets. The antibiotic Tetracycline is in clinical trials as an agent to make bone inhospitable to metastases, killing the cancer cells, stopping bone loss, and promoting the growth of healthy new bone tissue. Tetracycline inhibits the tumor cell from releasing the matrix metalloproteinase enzyme which breaks down bone and allows the tumor to expand. Take soy isoflavones at 100 to 150 mg daily, vitamin D3 at 800 I.U. or more daily, vitamin C, and the microcrystalline hydroxyapatite form of calcium.

PARANEOPLASTIC SYNDROMES
3 out of 4 cancer patients will experience a remote effect of the tumor.
1 in 5 has symptoms from tumor antigens and uncontrolled hormone output.

Tumors may produce parathyroid hormone (PTH), adrenocorticotrophic hormone (ACTH), thyroid stimulating hormone (TSH), or melanocyte stimulating hormone (MSH).

Multiple endocrine adenomatosis syndrome (MEA) can provoke galactorrhea (milk secretion) and gynecomastia (breast swelling).

Cutaneous (skin) manifestations could include purpura, flushing, erythema, phlebitis, urticaria, bullae, hyperpigmentation, pruritis, erythema nodosum, and shingles.

Neural (nerve) manifestations can be neuropathy, neuromyopathy, myopathy, myasthenia, progressive leukoencephalopathy, and seizures.

Blood cell production may shift from aplasia to erythrocythemia from ectopic erythropoietin, a hormone normally put out by the kidney to trigger the bone marrow to make red blood cells. Hemolysis may exacerbate anemia. Hyperviscosity - thickening of the blood - from globulin proteins or their clumping by cryoprecipitation may complicate syndromes of coagulation and fibrinolysis.

Kidney function can be compromised by ectopic antidiuretic hormone (ADH) produced by small cell lung cancer. Circulating immune complexes can inflame the kidneys, causing nephrotic syndrome.

Rheumatic arthritis is associated with lymphomas and ovarian cancer.

Amyloid starchy deposits can occur in any organ.

Endocarditis is associated with adenocarcinomas.

Arterial embolism triggers infarctions which can be fatal.

The carcinoid syndrome, as seen with small intestinal cancer, may cause endocardial fibrosis or bronchospastic pulmonary disease, diarrhea, abdomenal cramps, malabsorption, flushing due to serotonin excess. Monitor the urinary serotonin metabolite 5-HIAA.

Fever can exacerbate fatigue and malaise. Fever control will improve patient activity and vitality. However, a slight fever can also signal good immune activity.

Hypercalcemia can occur in squamous cell lung cancer, and very rarely also from tumor production of parathyroid hormone releasing protein (PTH-RP).

The bottom line with advanced cancer is that it is systemic - every part of the body becomes sick. Any new symptom in a cancer patient is significant and deserves investigation.

The cancer patient must be counselled against being unduly stoic or brave or macho about toughing out problems on their own - at least until they have been properly assessed, tested and diagnosed. We appreciate a fighting spirit, but only when backed up by a certainty of what we are fighting.

END-OF-LIFE ISSUES

The relief of pain and reduction of narcotics can help move a terminal patient into the death phase. Assisting a person to pass, and comforting the family, is an art that gives great satisfaction to a physician. There comes a time when everyone is willing to let go. There is joy in passing consciously and without fear.

The ethical decision to abandon curative therapy strategies for gentler palliative comfort-oriented care is a difficult one. The guiding principles are autonomy, nonmaleficence, beneficence and justice. Prudent decisions based on informed consent, fidelity to trust, compassion, integrity and temperance result in 'right and good' healing actions.

Homeopathics are very helpful in the emotional and mental transitions of palliative care, e.g. *Arsenicum album* 30C for late stage depression and anxiety. This remedy gives ease to the final moments of life.

Bach flower remedies are also great assists to the spirit and mind of the dying and the grieving.

Most physicians would be wise to study with hospice workers and call on them for support when the case is not realistically curable. Patients will often communicate their needs and problems more effectively to a non-physician. Whether it be legal advice on living wills and advanced directives, spiritual comfort, or allopathic pain control, palliation should be multidisciplinary and patient-directed.

Everyone wants to forestall death. We would prefer to die as young as possible, but as late as possible. I do place living at #1 on the list of priorities. However, those who experience at least the first stages of dying, such as cardiac arrest, who are later revived, all seem to have a pleasant experience. All lose their fear of death.

Spiritual beliefs alter a situation of loss of life into one of transition.
It is uncomfortable to be separated from a loved one by such an inalterable barrier. We lose contact, but a certain spirit lives on, even if only in the hearts of those loved ones who live on.

Death is not a failure for the patient, and it is not a failure for the health care team. It is condition we will all have. I have been honored and amazed to share births and deaths with my loved ones and with patients. These are experiences worth having, for they define BEING.

Chapter Nine -   NATUROPATHIC ONCOLOGY

The body has an innate gift for healing itself. It must be properly nourished, kept clean, and supported to do this job. Naturopathic medicines from all the healing traditions of the world are applied in a manner which respects the nature of the human being. Naturopathy is biologically sound, wholesome, and tailored to the individual patient. We have a physical body which is shaped by a genetic code inherited from forebears who had little problem with cancers, who ate a hunter-gatherer diet radically different from the modern diet, who inhabited an unpolluted world, and had a lot less stress. We have an emotional life, a discerning mind, and a spiritual dimension. Naturopathic medicine keeps these facts in focus in its healing process.

Every modern disease can be improved by gentle therapies which feed, harmonize, cleanse and balance the complex biological systems that synergize in great networks that make a whole person. We start with a sound diet of whole, living foods. We are what we eat. What else could we be made of? In all cases we want to reduce sugar and starches, increase protein, give good fats, increase fiber, and supply lots of antioxidants. Food concentrates, vitamins and minerals are important to shift the health rapidly in the face of aggressive disease. In this respect they are used as drugs. Later, as health returns, we can rely on dietetics alone. I cannot fathom doctors who think a few milligrams of this drug or that drug is all important, while the pounds of chemicals we take in as food are ignored as irrelevant.

We use medicinal as well as food plants, in as whole a form as possible, and in complex combinations to take advantage of the natural synergies that exist. Every living thing on this Earth is working with the same issues, the same stresses and problems, and many strategies have evolved to regulate growth and restore balance. We can integrate their successes into our biology to correct our health.

It is helpful to cleanse the body of parasites, fungi and harmful bacteria, and restore the friendly flora and fauna. We cleanse out the bowel and the blood. This controls inflammation and boosts immune competence. We use various gentle medicines which satisfy our committment to the Hippocratic Oath, to FIRST DO NO HARM. We cannot gain health just by cutting out disease. We respect the subtle and elegant power of the mind, of the immune system, and the homeostatic regulation in the body, and address all of them with medicines which are not necessarily cancer specifics. We are treating the person, not the disease.

I reiterate the primary strategies in naturopathic oncology:

- Improve nutrition and the terrain (the internal biochemical milieu)
- Remove promoters - clean up the chemicals and other pollutants in the home, workplace, environment, and especially the diet.
- Deal with toxic emotions, address fears and feelings, and practice positive attitudes and lifestyle.
- Reduce side-effects and symptoms of the disease and treatments.
- Support normal cell division
- Support differentiation of cells
- Stop mutation, stabilize the DNA genome
- Support DNA repair
- Support apoptosis - a built-in cellular program for natural removal of cells with unhealthy DNA, or cells no longer needed.
- Enhance cell-to-cell communication
- Control inflammation, cytokines and prostaglandins
- Support immune function, including removal of toxic fungi and parasites, control viral replication, restore the good flora and fauna of the gut.
- Anti-tumor medication - use synergies of non-toxic natural drugs
- Inhibit metastasis or spread
- Inhibit angiogenesis
- Detoxification
- Rejuvenation
- Prevent a reoccurrence of cancer.

DIAGNOSIS

Biopsy and histological evaluation are the only way to confirm cancer. It is unethical to offer to treat as cancer a case not medically confirmed, nor can one claim a cure until the positive test results are reversed.

- Cytology is a method of looking at loose cells taken off tumors or from around them. Pap smears, washings or brushings during endoscopies, and needle aspiration are alternatives to removing the primary tumor for evaluation.

- Supported by physical exam, scans, X-ray imaging, hormones, antigens, antibodies, neurological findings, tumor markers and tumor specific scans.

MEASURING RESPONSE TO THERAPY

<u>Complete response</u> - the disappearance of all evidence of tumor for at least 2 measurement periods separated by at least 4 weeks.

<u>Partial response</u> - a decrease of 50% or more in one or more measureable lesions with no progression of any lesion and no appearance of any new lesions for at least 4 weeks.

<u>Stable disease</u> - a decrease of less than 50% to an increase up to 25% in lesion diameter = no change

<u>Progression </u>- an increase of over 25% in diameter of a lesion or the appearance of any new lesions.

Do not persist with any treatment which does not produce clear evidence of a response in 2 to 4 weeks. Natural therapies may not act as fast as drugs, but they must act by this time frame or be abandoned. Most good outcomes begin with a response within a day or two.

ANALYZING A CANCER CASE

My naturopathic physician colleagues at the Cancer Treatment Centers of America have laid out a simple set of issues to explore with every new patient.
- What is the exact diagnosis?
- What is the stage of the disease? What is the natural history of that form of cancer at that stage - the average survival & prognosis? Develop realistic expectations, then strive to be an uncommon success.
- Why this person at this time with this disease? Disease has meaning, it is not random. Find the cause, physically, chemically, emotionally.
- What other medical conditions e.g. hypertension, diabetes, cardiovascular, immune, renal or liver complications?
- Nutritional status, digestion & absorption OK?
- Assess treatment options. Primary care, adjuncts, complementary care, palliation, social supports, psychological and self-healing assets.
- Get tumor markers before surgery!
- Follow-up with a regular screening program.
- Monitor lean body mass - BMI, serum albumen
- After treatment and recovery, detoxify & start a prevention program.

STANDARD OF CARE

Patients expect every type of physician to provide good care, even if the treatment is unorthodox or experimental.

- Always act in the patient's best interest. This means putting their welfare ahead of any desire for money, control, power, or another self-serving interest. I do not operate a crusade to convert people to natural medicine, and medical oncologists should not act as if they have all the answers either.
- Obtain informed consent. This basic legal principle means the patient needs to be told what the diagnosis is, what will happen without treatment, what all the treatment options are, and what the consequences of those choices will be. These must be explained in such a way that the patient actually understands them, and is able to give permission to the doctor without feeling pressured.
- Get involved early, act promptly, respond quickly.
- Tumor regression frequently occurs early in the course of effective treatment. If there is no objective evidence of a reasonable response to treatment in a few weeks, then new options must be examined, or a referral made to another practitioner for exploration of other options
- Assess every 3 months for the first year, every 6 months in the second year, and annually thereafter. Usually after 5 years cancer free the patient is considered 'cured'. The odds of reoccurrence fall off sharply by that time.

SUMMARY OF THE ACTION OF KEY NATURAL COMPOUNDS

APOPTOSIS PROMOTERS - quercitin, curcumin, mistletoe, green tea EGCG, betulinic acid, caffeine, genestein, berberine, vitamin E succinate, glutathione, N-acetyl cysteine, catechin, cayenne. Noscapine from the poppy *Papaver somniferum*.

ANTI-METASTATICS - fractionated citrus pectin, heparin, larch arabinogalactan, aloe vera juice, EPA omega 3 oils, CLA, bromelain.

ANTI-ANGIOGENICS - catechin, EGCG, curcumin, vitamins A, D & E, shikonin, genestein and shark liver oil. See also COX-2 inhibitors. Sodium chromoglycolate.

INDUCERS OF DIFFERENTIATION - butyrate, berberine, bromelain, retinoids, vitamins A & D, quercitin, calcium. Burdock root and parsley inhibit mutations.

PROTEIN KINASE SIGNAL INHIBITORS - curcumin, genestein, green tea EGCG, milk thistle, vitamin E succinate (VES).

HEAT SHOCK PROTEIN BLOCKERS - quercitin, alpha lipoic acid

CELL-TO-CELL COMMUNICATION MODIFIERS - GLA, CLA, bromelain, green tea catechins (EGCG), melatonin, integrins.

TNF INHIBITORS - melatonin, milk thistle, cat's claw, VES, genestein, EGCG.

COX-2 INHIBITORS - scutellaria, feverfew, rosemary, curcumin, ginger, isatis tinctoria, propolis & CAPE, vitamin A, grapeseed proanthocyanins, green tea EGCG, licorice, garlic, bromelain and cold-water fish oils.

CYTOTOXICS - berberine, mistletoe, graviola, carnivora, isatis, yew bark.

IMMUNE MODULATORS - astragalus, ligusticum, maitake, shiitake, ganoderma, plant sterols & sterolins, Bu Zhong Yi Qi Tang, Shih Chuan Da Bu Wan, ashwagandha. Proteolytics: bromelain, pancreatin, proteases. *Polyerga* spleen peptides and thymus extracts. Alkylglycerols from shark liver oil and omega 3 fats from cod liver oil. Larch arabinogalactan, Echinacea, Panax ginseng, Panax notoginseng, curcumin, cat's claw and Saposhnikovia divaricata. *Iscador* injectable mistletoe extract. MRV, MBV and BCG vaccines. Cimetidine 800-1000 mg.

TOPOISOMERASE INHIBITORS - green tea (I), boswellia (I & II), berberine (I & II), camptothecin, etoposide.

ANTI-CACHEXICS - EPA omega 3 oils, CLA, melatonin, vitamin E, green tea EGCG, cat's claw, milk thistle, *Ukrain*.

HORMONE MODULATORS - flaxseed, melatonin, indole 3 carbinol (I3C), diindolylmethane (DIM), potassium iodide.

ANTI-VIRALS - *Engystol, Thymuline*, echinacea, lomatia, graviola, vitamin A, vitamin C, glutathione, Newcastle paramyxovirus nasal spray.

ANTI-PARASITICS - Flaxseed, psyllium husks, graviola, berberine.

p53 GENE MODULATORS - phytic acid (IP6), N-acetyl-cysteine, quercitin, melatonin, catechin, green tea EGCG, grapeseed OPC's, vitamin E, antioxidants.

CORE NATUROPATHIC THERAPIES IN CANCER

A cancer patient needs emotional support first. When they are ready to take responsibility for their own life, they can make life-saving changes to their lifestyle. The diet must be made clean and wholesome. Exercise, relaxation, stress management and other self-care therapies need to become part of their routine.

A primary set of remedies to arrest neoplasia and reduce the risk of spread are the bioflavenoids:

- *green tea* extract with 95% polyphenols: 500 mg three times daily
- *curcumin*: 500 mg three times daily
- *grapeseed* standardized OPC extract: 100 mg three times daily

These must be given together. They are quite remarkable, and universally applicable. Often early cancers stop growing and spreading.

Other important front-line medicines usually considered are:

- melatonin: 10 to 20 mg at bedtime only
- potassuim iodide: 1 to 2 capsules daily
- cod liver oil: 1 to 2 Tablespoons daily for vit. A & D, EPA & DHA
- quercitin: 500 mg three times daily
- vitamin E: 800 to 1,200 I.U. - succinate form is best (VES)
- vitamin C: 2,000 to 3,000 mg, with supporting antioxidants selenium, N-acetyl cysteine, glutathione and alpha-lipoic acid
- sterols and sterolins: 1 capsule three times daily away from food.
- butyrate: 3 grams three times daily with meals
- proteolytic enzymes ad lib (use freely)
- ImmunoCal *HMS 90* whey protein isolate
- Hoxsey tincture with homeopathic nosodes: 25 to 30 drops three times daily, in a little water, sip slowly. No food or drink for 15 minutes.
- Yunnan Baiyao or *Panax pseudoginseng var. notoginseng.*
- Ping Xiao Pian, Anticancerlin, Canelim or Internal Dissolution Pills.

To rid parasites and toxins:

- flaxseed: 1 to 2 Tablespoons daily
- graviola leaf: 3 capsules up to 3 times daily
- *Herbotox*: 1 capsule twice daily
- *Para-Sit* cleanse: 2 capsules three times daily
- milk thistle

For immune support:
- vaccines - BCG, MRV, *C. parvum, Respivax* or *Polyvaccinum*
- Mushroom glucans - Reishi, Maitake MD, PSK or PSP, shiitake, AHCC
- homeopathics *Engystol* and *Thymuline.*
- Histamine
- *Polyerga* spleen peptides, thymus glandular extract.
- Vitamin C, Vitamin A, zinc and selenium

To inhibit spread:
- modified citrus pectin or larch arabinogalactans
- aloe vera juice
- vitamin C
- bromelain

For general good health:
- exercise
- rest
- play
- probiotics to balance gut bacterial flora
- take a good 1-a-day multivitamin high in B-complex & minerals
- extra fiber such as psyllium husks with fresh-ground flaxseed
- follow the basic cancer diet and prevention strategies
- follow the Law of Attraction to get what you need from Creator.

In very advanced cancers we would usually add one of:
- *Iscador* mistletoe injections
- *Ukrain* injection
- *Careseng* ginseng intravenously & orally
- megadoses of vitamin C intravenously and orally

The following chapters describe further steps which can be added for specific cancer types. Work with your own wisdom and the style of the practitioners on your team to individualize your cancer survival program.

Chapter Ten -   INTEGRATIVE CARE OF BREAST CANCER

EPIDEMIOLOGY

The most common cancer of women in North America is breast cancer. Risk in Asia and Africa is 4 to 5 times less. 1% of breast cancer cases are male. Approximately one woman in 8 in North America will develop this disease in her lifetime. Before 1971 the risk was 1 in 20! It is the second leading cause of death in American women, and the leading cause of death in the age group 40 to 55 years. The death rate has been unchanged from 1920 to 1990. We are not really 'winning the war' on this cancer!

Breast cancer cells have an average doubling time of about 100 days, which is relatively slow. There is time to reflect and decide among the various treatment options.

RISK FACTORS FOR DEVELOPING BREAST CANCER

- Family history in first degree relative - mother or sister
- Early menarche (start of menstruation)
- Late onset of menopause
- Estrogen excess such as estrogen replacement therapy in menopause or use of birth control pills before age 35 or longer than

5 years. Estrogen and progesterone combination hormone replacement therapy (HRT) is also linked to increased risk of gallbladder cancer, stroke, heart attack, blood clots and Alzheimer's

- Obesity - fat cells make estrogen via aromatase enzyme
- High fat diet, especially those high in arachidonic acid and saturated fat.
- Moderate to high alcohol consumption increases risk 50 to 100%Risk is entirely dose-dependent - for example, risk increases 45 to 50% with consumption of more than half of a glass of wine daily! Steven Bowlin of Case Western Reserve University states that 25% of breast cancers can be attributed to alcohol.
- Nulliparous – never having a child – risk up 30%
- Child-bearing after age 30. First full term pregnancy after 25 puts up risk 40% over those having a child before 20.
- Excess exposure to xenobiotics with estrogenic properties such as pesticides and herbicides. For example organochlorine pesticides like DDT increase risk of larger and more agressive cancers.
- Exposure to anti-psychotic drugs which are dopamine antagonists, and anti-emetic dopamine antagonists for vomiting, because they elevate prolactin.

GENETIC FACTORS IN BREAST CANCER

- Genetic factors may only cause 5% of cases. Jewish people have slightly higher risk than other races.

- BRCA1 gene on chromosome 17 normally repairs DNA damage independent of p53. Female carriers of mutated BRCA1 have an 85% lifetime risk of breast and up to 50% risk of ovarian cancers. Male carriers have 4X increased risk of developing colon cancer, and 3X increased risk of developing prostate cancer. BRAC1 breast tumors are very sensitive to chemotherapy, with extremely high rates of tumor and axillary (lymph nodes in the armpit) clearance, particularly with anthracycline drugs.

- BRCA2 gene on chromosome 13 is associated with increased risk of early onset breast cancer, and 4 times increased risk of uterine cancer. Carriers of BRAC mutations tend to have tumors with higher grades, more necrosis, and more proliferative activity. Male carriers have 15 times increased risk of breast cancer and 4 times increased risk of early prostate cancer.

- The p53 tumor suppressor gene is altered in about 50% of cases of advanced metastatic disease.

- Reduced p27 levels in the nucleus correlate with tumor aggressiveness and poor survival. P27 is a direct inhibitor of cyclin-dependent kinase 2 (cdk2) responsible for transcription factors that promote DNA replication. In advanced breast cancer a protein kinase Akt bars p27 from the nucleus by phosphorylating p27 in its nuclear localization signal sector. Phosphorylated P27 ends up sequestered in the cytoplasm, unable to bind up and inhibit the nuclear protein cdk2 involved in cell regulation. Akt also fosters cell proliferation, survival and motility through P13K kinase which is activated by the HER2 and epidermal growth factor receptors.

- Her-2/neu gene overexpression or amplification results in increased increased HER-2/neu protein, which results in overexpression of EGFRs - epitheliod growth factor receptors. This is particularly problematic in rapidly proliferating tumors. There is also speculation this gene may reduce estrogen and progesterone hormone receptors on the surface of the breast cancer cells making them harder to cure.

Once breast cancer has occurred, the risk of a second occurrence goes up 5 fold. A person with breast cancer is also at higher than average risk of developing cancer of the colon, ovaries or endometrium of the uterus (lining of the womb).

REDUCING RISK OF BREAST CANCER

- High intake of dietary fiber, vitamin C, betacarotene, lycopenes, legumes, cruciferous vegetables, green tea.

- Dietary phytoestrogens such as soy foods.

- Low fat diet, to 20% of calories as fat. Monosaturates such as oleic acid in canola oil and olive oil are protective. Omega 3 fatty acids are protective, as found in wild salmon, tuna, halibut, mackerel, sardines and herring; also in nuts and seeds.

- Regular physical exercise, at least 30 minutes aerobic exercise three times a week.

- Sunshine and vitamin D. So many people are avoiding sun exposure and using sunscreens to reduce risk of skin cancers, but now many Canadians are showing up with vitamin D deficiency, particularly in winter.

- Breastfeeding helps - the longer the better, for you and for your baby. The breast tissue completes its differentiation and carcinogens are eliminated in the breast milk. The months during pregnancy without periods also are risk reducers, so more kids and more nursing in the past may have helped keep rates lower.

- Stress management to moderate cortisol and blood sugar fluctuations.

- Avoid use of anti-perspirants. I like to use natural grapefruit seed extract (GSE) deodorants.

- Maintain good bowel bacteria with enteric-coated probiotics.

- Avoid alcohol, but if you must drink, take folate and vitamin B6.

- Detoxify your body of xenobiotics with an annual body cleanse.
  A naturopathic physician can guide you as to diet and herbs appropriate for your health. We can avoid a lot of risk by eating organic food, choosing natural hygiene and cleaning products, and generally reducing our reliance on synthetic chemical products in our homes.

DIAGNOSIS & SCREENING

Breast Self Exam - recent studies suggest BSE may not be able to detect cancer early enough to alter the clinical outcome. However, many women prefer to be proactive, and recognize that 7 to 10% of palpable masses will be missed by a mammogram. The smallest palpable mass is about 8 millimeters in diameter, which would contain about a billion cancer cells at about three fourths of their lifespan in age. Perform BSE 5 to 7 days after menses, every month. Cancer can occur soon after a 'normal' mammogram. Watch for a persisitent rash on the nipple, which may be the only warning of Paget's disease.

Physical Exam by a Physician or Nurse - professional PE should be done every 3 years between ages 20 - 40, and every 2 years thereafter. All palpable lesions should be biopsied. Most will not be malignant.

Mammography - expert opinion about the value of mammograms has changed several times in living memory. About 0.3% of asymptomatic Canadian adult women may harbor breast cancer. The current consensus is that they are probably helpful at early detection for women over age 50. Swedish studies on women ages 48 - 69 showed up to 45% reduced mortality from breast cancer. Modern mammograms use a very low dose of radiation, in the standard two view bilateral test. There is a potential to detect masses under 5 mm diameter. The pathognomic (characteristic) lesion is a high attenuation mass with spiculated margins. There is a false negative rate of 10 to 30%! This can be from the mass being hidden in dense breast tissue, interpretive error, and because the entire breast is not imaged. Mammography can detect about 69% of cancers (sensitivity) and misdiagnose about 16% of cases (specificity).
95% of masses found by screening mammography are benign, but all should be carefully evaluated.

Miraluma, Mibi and Scintigraphy - mibi scans are widely used in coronary disease assessment, and have been adapted for use in breast cancer diagnosis. The mibi scan uses an IV injection of approximately 1000 MBq of sesamibi isotope (technectium-99m hexakis 2-methoxyisonitrile) into a fasting patient who has avoided caffeine and other vasoconstrictors. The patient rests prone, breasts hanging down through openings in the table, so there is no compression applied to the breast. The mibi isotope accumulates in mitochondria, and measures metabolic activity. The original protocol called a Miraluma scan had approximately the same utility as mammograms. However, recently the BEST scan system has added high-dose dipyridamole (HDD) to vasodilate and enhance isotope uptake. This produces accurate discrimination of normal breast tissue from inflammation, and detects early cancers as small as 4mm diameter.

Ultrasound - Diagnostic ultrasound is not useful for screening, but will determine with 100% accuracy if a lesion is a cyst or a solid mass.
It can augment mammography when breast tissue is very dense.

Magnetic Resonance Imaging - MRI's will not show calcifications, but will show vascularity and can therefore discriminate a local recurrence in a surgical scar. Also it is a more sensitive test for bone metastases than a bone scan.

Thermography - very sensitive infrared cameras are being used to detect hot spots in the body, especially in the breast, which can indicate malignant changes in tissue including angiogenesis, as well as inflammation. Thermal scans easily discriminate fibrocystic lumps, as they have no thermal signature. Hot areas can be found as much as 3 years before a cancer is diagnosable, making preventative care a reality.
The Bales Scientific thermal image processor is a refinement which allows images to be taken in a room that is not cold, as required for earlier scanners. Not only is this more comfortable, but after a baseline image is taken, cold air may be blown onto the breast, provoking a sympathetic nervous system response to cold stress. Normal tissue will undergo vasoconstriction and show up as cooler, but areas of new blood vessel growth - angiogenesis - will not cool.

BIOPSY

FINE NEEDLE ASPIRATION - is frequently employed, although the technique has a 5% failure rate. Ultrasound or computerized stereotactic (3D) guidance is sometimes used, mainly for non-palpable lesions.

EXCISIONAL BIOPSY - more invasive, but more reliable.Invasion of the tumor into the margins of the biopsy sample indicates it has not been completely removed, and indicates a more aggressive tumor.

LYMPH NODE DISSECTION - samples the lymph nodes, such as those in the armpit, for cancer spreading from the lateral breast through the tail of the breast. Breast tumors of 1 cm diameter can produce cancerous tumors able to live in the lymphatic nodes. Lymph node positive status indicates the spread of the cancer regionally in the body, which increases the risk the cancer can form metastatic colonies in distant sites. Removing these cancerous lymph nodes reduces the risk of a local reoccurence of the cancer in the nodes, but it does not reduce the risk of reoccurence of the cancer in the breast or at distant metastatic sites. The latter are generally aggressive, treatment resistant, and often fatal. Unfortunately, local control achieved by lymph node dissection does not increase life expectancy.

Lymph node involvement is not as ominous as distant metastases, and women who are node-positive frequently can live out a full lifespan. Node positive premenopausal women clearly benefit from chemotherapy. Node negative premenopausal women benefit less from chemotherapy.

Breast carcinoma cells in a lymph node are stimulated to grow - independent of anchorage - by stromal cells production of the major mitogens IGF-1 and EGF.

SENTINEL NODE BIOPSY - A more conservative approach to node status, it involves the injection of a blue dye or a radioactive tracer at the tumor, and removal of the first lymph node the dye or tracer drains to. This can eliminate "strip-mining" the whole lymphatic chain, which has a high incidence of lymphedema and other morbidity. Removing lymph nodes does not improve the length of time patient will survive.

MAMMASTATIN - mammastatin serum assay (MSA) is a screening blood test for breast cancer risk developed in 1998 at the University of Michigan. It has application similar to PSA testing for prostate cancer. Overall accuracy is about 85%. High levels of the protein marker would normally be followed with a mammogram and/or genetic screening.

GRADING & PROGNOSTIC INDICATORS

Scarff-Bloom-Richardson (SBR) classification - scores the mitotic rate, nuclear pleomorphism and tubule formation seen by microscope.
   Grade I: 3 – 5 points = well differentiated
   Grade II: 6 – 7 points = moderately differentiated
   Grade III: 8 – 9 points = poorly differentiated.

Histological grade - rates the tissue on how much normal cellular architecture such as ductal structures are preserved.
   Grade I: well differentiated
   Grade II: moderately differentiated
   Grade III: poorly differentiated.

STAGING

Staging may be by the TNM surgical rating system (see page 23), or by the clinical staging system:

             Stage 0   = intraductal cancer in situ
             Stage I   = small tumor under 2 cm with no + nodes
             Stage II   = medium tumor 2 - 5 cm with + axillary lymph node
             Stage IIIA = large tumor over 5 cm with palpable axillary node
             Stage IIIB = tumor of any size with extension into the chest
                        wall, skin or internal mammary lymphatic chain
             Stage IV = distant metastases and invasion into the chest wall.

MENOPAUSAL STATUS: #1 prognostic factor, breast cancer occurring before menopause is exposed to more estrogen, and tends to be much more dangerous.

LYMPH NODE STATUS: #2 prognostic factor, + or - for metastasis. Tumors in the medial breast spread into the thoracic and mediastinal lymph nodes, while from the lateral breast they spread into the axillary lymph chains. Negative lymph node patients have a 70% cure rate with surgery and radiation. Only 1 in 3 of those who will have a recurrence will be helped with subsequent chemotherapy. Positive lymph node status will have under 50% survival with surgery and radiation alone.

S-PHASE: cell cycle analysis, looks at the proportion of cells in S-phase where new DNA is being synthesized in preparation for the division of a tumor cell into two cells. Higher values mean the tumor is growing more rapidly. In breast cancer the S-phase count can range from 1 to 20%,; values over 7% give a poorer prognosis.

ESTROGEN RECEPTOR STATUS: ER+ or ER- determines the tumor sensitivity to hormone therapy. ER+ has a better prognosis, as the cells are more normal.

PROGESTERONE RECEPTOR STATUS: PR+ or PR-. PR+ may have a significantly better prognosis. It is believed that ER-/PR+ represents a false negative ER result and that ER+/PR- represents a false positive ER result as PR is a product of an intact estrogen-ER pathway, thus PR+ is only possible if ER is also expressed.

IMMUNOHISTOCHEMISTRY: includes the detection of abnormal tumor proteins such as HER-2/neu receptors, also called C-erb-B2 receptors, for both epidermal and platelet-derived growth factors. These receptors are over-expressed in some breast comedo type ductal carcinoma in situ (DCIS), ovarian, lung, prostate, and stomach cancers. Associated with earlier relapses and poorer prognosis.

DNA PLOIDY: uses flow cytometry techniques to look for multiple sets of chromosomes representing cells in mitotoic division, giving an average value for the amount of DNA in the tumor cells. Abnormal DNA content strongly correlates with the aggressiveness of the tumor. Aneuploidy corresponds to poorly differentiated tumors.

TUMOR MARKERS: CEA, CA-125, CA 15-3, CA 549, CA M26, CA M29, CA 27.29, MCA, PSA, isoferritin, tissue polypeptide antigen (TPA), mammary tumor-associated glycoprotein, kappa casein.

CYCLIN E: in truncated isoforms in high amounts in tumors, as measured by the Western blot test, predicts high risk of reoccurrence and poorer survival. Australian doctors say over-expression of this regulator of the transition from G1 to S phase in the cell cycle is the most powerful predictor of breast cancer outcome.

BREAST CANCER TYPES

DUCTAL CARCINOMA IN SITU (DCIS) - is the proliferation of cancer within the milk ducts without any invasion through the basement membrane. The cancer is unicentric within a segment, and is found in occult form in about 30% of females autopsied. On mammograms DCIS will typically show microcalcifications.
Pure ductal carcinoma in situ rarely metastasizes, so if the lesion is removed with the margins of the sample free of disease, sentinel node biopsy is optional. The most common form is non-comedo cribriform type. Mastectomy has a 98% cure rate. Lumpectomy has up to 60% failure rate, with half of the recurrences being invasive carcinoma. Radiation may improve control after lumpectomy.
COMEDO VARIANT tends to high nuclear grade (80% are aneuploid) and necrosis, ER-, and highly over-expressing HER/neu+. The comedo type is more aggressive, has a worse prognosis, and warrants prompt and aggressive treatment.

LOBULAR CARCINOMA IN SITU (LCIS) - is multicentric cancer within multiple breast lobules, which never produces a mass that can be detected by mammography. Risk of occurrence in the other breast is 10 to 25%. About 37% will develop invasive cancer in either breast, with risk increasing by about 1% per year. The standard approach is bilateral mastectomy with immediate reconstructive surgery, never chemo or radiation.

INFILTRATING DUCTAL CARCINOMA (IDC) - represents 75% of all breast tumors. More frequently metastatic to bone, lung and liver.

INFILTRATING LOBULAR CARCINOMA (ILC) - up to 10% of breast cancers are ILC, with a tendency to metastasize to the meninges causing carcinomatous meningitis, to the eyes, ovaries, retroperitoneum and serosal surfaces, causing intestinal or urethral obstruction.

TUBULAR CARCINOMA (TC) - About 2% of breast cancers, tend to be well differentiated, rarely metastasize to the axilla, and typically ER+ and PR+.

MEDULLARY CARCINOMA (MC) - About 6% of breast cancers, occurring at younger ages, often metastasizing locally, producing large axillary nodes, and typically ER+, PR-, p53+

INFLAMMATORY BREAST CANCER (IBC) - Accounts for 1% of breast cancers, the most aggressive type, with the poorest prognosis. 1 in 4 cases will have pain in the breast or nipple. There is rapid onset of symptoms, 90% probability of axillary lymph node involvement, progression to stage IIIB, typically ER- and PR-, and up to 50% risk of contralateral breast cancer.

SURGERY

- Lumpectomy - tumor removed with at least a 1 cm margin of healthy tissue.
- Quadrantectomy - tumor removed with a 3 cm margin and the overlying skin and underlying fascia.
- Modified radical mastectomy - removal of the entire breast
- Radical Mastectomy - removal of the breast and underlying muscle and associated tissues. Radical mastectomy is not associated with better long-term survival than less extensive surgery, and so has been largely abandoned. NSABP in Pittsburgh published 5 and 10 year follow-up results, and now 25 year follow-up shows the same result.
- Mastectomy is generally contraindicated if there are distant metastases. Removing the larger tumor can de-inhibit growth of metastases.
- In premenopausal women it is critical to do the surgery during the luteal phase of the menstrual cycle. The high progesterone levels at this time lowers the potent angiogenesis stimulator vascular endothelial growth factor (VEGF), and is associated with much longer survival times. For example, serum progesterone at least 4 mcg/ml corresponded to 65% survival at 18 years post-surgery versus 35% for those with lower progesterone.

For small cancers under 1 cm. the standard of care is lumpectomy followed by radiation, and if ER+ Tamoxifen may be considered. The radiation doubles the chances of avoiding a relapse (local radiation after lumpectomy or breast-conserving surgery for early stage primary breast cancer will decrease 20 year rates of recurrence of cancer in that breast to about 14%, compared to about 39% with the surgery alone, regardless of node status.

Breast surgery, node biopsies and radiation therapy can ablate and scar lymphatic drainage of the arm via the axilla, causing lymphedema.
See Chapter 9: Complications & Emergencies - Lymphedema, p 136.

Ovarian Ablation - removal of the ovaries by surgery (oophorectomy) or their destruction by chemotherapy or radiation removes estrogen stimulation and is associated with improved survival. Premenopausal women with highly ER positive (over 20) tumors may benefit from ovarian ablation more than they can benefit from chemotherapy.

HORMONE BLOCKADE

Hormone blockade will starve tumors of promoting factors but resistance commonly develops in 5 to 6 years. General side-effects can include hot flashes, impotence, reduced libido, breast enlargement, accelerated bone loss & osteoporosis, muscle weakness, muscle wasting, liver damage, reduced night vision, nausea, diarrhea, alcohol intolerance. Patients also show increased rates of death from cardiovascular disease, stroke, and infection

Tamoxifen - a selective estrogen receptor modulator (SERM) with estrogen antagonist and partial estrogen agonist effects. It is widely used for any breast cancer with ER+ status, for those with spread into the lymph nodes and especially for post-menopausal women. It may also benefit ER- cases, but at 3 to 10 fold less benefit than ER+ cases. It is not well indicated in pre-menopausal breast cancer.
The estrogen receptor co-activator AIB-1 gene product amplifies estrogen and Tamoxifen's estrogen agonist effect. AIB-1 is in turn amplified by HER-2. It has been found that AIB-1 positive / HER-2 positive patients seem not to be helped by adjuvant tamoxifen, and in fact may be harmed by it. HER-1 and HER-2 are related to epidermal growth factor receptors as well as modulating estrogen receptors.
Tamoxifen also increases sex hormone binding globulins (SHBG), decreases IGF, and can reduce TGF alpha. Other benefits: increased bone mass, reduced risk of heart disease, and slightly reduced risk of contralateral breast cancer (the usual 8% occurrence is brought down to 5%).

However, the contralateral tumors that do occur tend to be ER- (27% with Tamoxifen vs. 4% without the drug) which are harder to treat. Side-effects include blood clots, hot flashes, vaginal dryness or discharge, irregular menses, toxicity to the eyes with visual impairment, depression, poor concentration, asthma, and increased risk of liver cancer. The risk of endometrial cancer is increased by 2 to 3 fold, and requires annual screening tests. Report any changes in your health to your physician and get annual eye and physical exams as a minimum.

Contraindications include macular degeneration or a history of thrombo-embolic disease. Do not take Tamoxifen with birth control pills.

Tamoxifen combined with Goserelin is superior in safety and in reducing reoccurrence compared to standard chemotherapy drugs like cyclophosphamide, methotrexate and fluorouracil in stage I or II premenopausal hormone responsive breast cancer. These patients first have surgery to reduce the tumor burden.

....

Other hormone blocker drugs include Lupron and Zoladex, analogues of luteinizing hormone releasing hormone (LHRH). These have significant risks of thrombo-embolism and pulmonary embolism.
LHRH agonists can cause a flare reaction as hormones spike up, then fall. This aggravation can be spared by taking an anti-androgen for one week prior to this therapy. Soy isoflavones may ameliorate many of the adverse effects of these drugs, such as bone loss.

Megace is synthetic progestin, antagonistic to estrogen.

Casodex and Eulixen are anti-androgens.

Fulvestrant is a new class of anti-estrogen completely free of agonist activity. When breast cancer progresses despite Tamoxifen and aromatase inhibitors, this second-line drug will stabilize the disease and provide partial responses. Side effects can include fatigue, nausea and vomiting, chills, constipation, hot flashes and stomatitis.

AROMATASE INHIBITORS

Aromatase inhibitors block the enzyme estrogen synthetase which converts androgens or male hormones into estrogens or female hormones. Androstenedione is converted into estrone and testosterone into estradiol. This can occur in the liver, fatty tissue, muscle, skin, breast and breast tumors.

Aromatase inhibitors are not effective in premenopausal women, as they cannot overcome other hormone sources such as the ovaries.

The third generation oral aromatase inhibitors suppress circulating estrogen by 80 to 90%. These include the reversible nonsteroidal agents Anastrozole and Letrozole, and the irreversible steroidal inhibitor Exemestane. They are becoming popular for patients with ER+ tamoxifen refractory metastatic breast cancer. Time to disease progression is similar to tamoxifen therapy. Menopausal symptoms occur, but are less severe than with tamoxifen, other than increased bone loss. There is also a signifigant reduction in the incidence of contralateral breast cancer, and a small reduction in distant metastases and endometrial cancer.

Aromatase inhibitors may be used in ER+ early stage postmenopausal breast cancer, especially in those intolerant of Tamoxifen, or concerned about thromboembolic risk. It is not recommended for persons at high risk of osteopenia or osteoporosis (bone loss).

Quercitin is a natural aromatase inhibitor.

Remember COX-2 inhibitors block prostaglandins which promote the expression of the aromatase gene CYP19. These may well produce a nice synergy with quercitin. My clinical experience with such combination has been positive.

CHEMOTHERAPY

Chemotherapy is NOT justified for patients who are node negative and also have:

- tumors 1 cm or smaller
- tumors 1 to 2 cm with favorable indicators like ER+ status and a good histological grade.
- tumors with a low fatality rate such as tubular, colloid, mucinous or papillary forms.

Examples of common protocols :

- CMF – cytoxan, methotrexate and 5-fluorouracil
- FAC – 5-FU, adriamycin and cyclophosphamide
- TAC – taxol, adriamycin and cyclophosphamide
- AC – adriamycin and cytoxan
- Chemo + Herceptin monoclonal antibodies

Herceptin is a humanized anti-HER2 monoclonal antibody which binds to trans-membrane growth factor receptors. These receptors bind to EGF and PDGF and activate tyrosine kinase activity inside the cells.

High dose taxanes, bone marrow autologous transplantation and extended courses of chemotherapy have not yielded improved survival. It is best to use combinations of drugs to reduce toxicities, and not space the treatments out - a "dose-dense" approach is preferred.

A promising new agent being studied is the farnesyl transferase inhibitor (FTI) R115777, which has induced remissions or prolonged disease stabilization in 25% of advanced breast cancer cases refractory to chemo or hormone blockade. Myelosuppression is less with intermittent dosing than continuous infusions. FTI's inhibit the oncogene ras pathway, a guanine nucleotide binding protein which functions upstream of one of the main signal transduction pathways controlling cell proliferation, morphology, stress response and survival. Ras is activated when bound to the plasma membrane, which is mediated by a post-translational modification known as farnesylation. The FTI may shift processing of Rho-B to an inactivated geranylated state, rather than the active farnesylated state.

ALTERNATIVE & COMPLEMENTARY REMEDIES FOR BREAST CANCER

GAMMA LINOLENIC ACID (GLA) - 2.8 grams or 8 capsules of evening primrose oil (EPO) daily gives a faster clinical response to Tamoxifen. GLA produces anti-inflammatory prostaglandins.

MELATONIN - is highly synergistic with Tamoxifen, at doses of 10 to 20 mg at bedtime. Melatonin down-regulates estrogen receptors, reduces circulating estrogen and prolactin, suppresses tumor fatty acid uptake, and blocks estrogen and epidermal growth factors.

FLAXSEED LIGNANS - from 2 tablespoons ground flaxseed daily have been shown to reduce the rate of growth of breast tumors, and is significantly effective at preventing the spread of breast cancer.   Flaxseed binds estrogen in the bowel, preventing re-uptake, and stimulates production of sex hormone binding globulins (SHBG's), removing hormones from the bloodstream. Flaxseed works best with a low fat diet high in other lignan fibre from fruit, berries, vegetables, legumes, and whole grains.

SOY FOODS - highly protective diets yield about 150 mg daily of soy isoflavones. Compounds such as genistein and daidzein in soy are anti-angiogenic, antioxidant, induce cell differentiation, decrease luteinizing hormone (LH) and follicle stimulating hormone (FSH). Dietary phytoestrogens are anti-estrogenic, competing with estradiol for the type II estrogen binding sites. 60 grams of soy foods can yield 45 mg of isoflavones, which could match the effects of Tamoxifen.

INDOLES - indole-3-carbinol (I3C), from the cabbage family of vegetables, converts 16-hydroxyestrogens to 2-hydroxy forms. 16-OH-estrone is highly estrogenic and initiates carcinogenic DNA damage. It is associated with obesity. The safer 2-OH forms of estrone and estradiol are increased by aerobic exercise, green tea, licorice, I3C, DIM, and the cabbage family vegetables. It is interesting to note that the famous physician Galen prescribed cabbage leaf poultices for breast cancer 2,000 years ago.
I3C is anti-estrogenic, negatively modulates estrogen receptor transcription, and suppresses breast cancer invasion and migration.

OMEGA 3 OILS - flaxseed and other omega 3 oils, such as fish, seal and walnut oils, reduce rates of metastasis. These also thin the blood, and must be used with caution around surgery or with blood thinning medications.

VITAMIN D - 1,25-dihydroxy D3, a fat-soluble vitamin activated by sunlight on the skin, inhibits IGF-signaling and associated growth stimulation of breast cancer cells, promotes apoptosis, and may have anti-estrogenic activity. *D induces Differentiation.*

GREEN TEA - green tea polyphenols induce apoptosis in breast cancer cells. They are free radical scavengers. EGCG inhibits urokinase, an enzyme involved in tumor invasion and metastasis.

QUERCITIN - this bioflavenoid is an aromatase inhibitor, reducing estrogen production from fat cells. Use with bromelain for better absorption. Consider adding COX II inhibitors.

VITEX – *Vitex agnes castus* or chaste tree berry lowers prolactin (PL) levels, increases progesterone, decreases estrogen, lowers follicle-stimulating hormone (FSH) and raises luteinizing hormone (LH).

VITAMIN B6 - at 150 mg daily reduces prolactin levels.

VITAMIN E - antioxidant for fatty tissue, regulates hormones, heals damaged tissue.

MILK THISTLE - inhibits or modulates epidermal growth factor EGF, active in all carcinomas. Regulating EGF may be useful in modulating related estrogen receptors. This wonderful herb protects and detoxifies the liver.

Other breast cancer adjuncts -
- lycopene - including stewed tomatoes
- mixed natural carotenoids - the colored fruits and vegetables
- folic acid - green leafy vegetables
- vitamin A - green leafy vegetables
- rosemary - a delightful spice which harmonizes hormones

Constrained liver chi is the start of a causal chain which leads to all tumors and lumps. Its cause is often in the emotions, such as frustration, resentment, anger - especially when these are repressed and internalized.
Learning to express what you really feel is a key to true health.

Chapter Eleven - INTEGRATIVE CARE OF PROSTATE CANCER

EPIDEMIOLOGY

Prostate cancer is very common in developed countries. In the United States, 1 man in 6 will develop invasive prostate cancer in his lifetime. 1 in 4 African-Americans will develop prostate cancer, a rate of 137 per 100,000 population.   In Europe and South America the rate of incidence is 20 to 50 per 100,000. In China the rate is only 2.3 per 100,000.

Key risk factors:
- high fat diet, especially saturated fats.
- hormone exposure
- xenobiotics such as pesticides, herbicides and fertilizers
- heavy metals such as cadmium
- smoking tobacco
- family history of prostate cancer
- being married - but a good marriage reduces other risks.

The role of pesticides remains controversial - to apologists for the chemical industry. A Danish study showed the highest incidence among farmers - but the lowest incidence was among organic farmers. Recent evidence points to many pesticides and herbicides acting like estrogen in the body. Estrogen receptors in prostate tissue control expression of the telomerase gene hTERT. Increased telomerase activity marks the early stages of prostate cancer. Telomerase mRNA increases 2 to 3 fold with induction of estrogen receptors alpha & beta, up-regulating gene transcription and thus cell growth. ER alpha expression increases during the progression of prostate cancer.

The cancer gene bcl-2 is active in maintaining prostate cancers.
The gene bcl-6 also plays a role in prostate cancer.

A very large study is now underway to determine the role of vitamin E and selenium in preventing prostate cancer. The SELECT study by the National Cancer Institute (NCI) and Southwest Oncology Group will run for 12 years, follow 32,400 patients in Canada, USA and Puerto Rico. Participants must have no sign of prostate cancer at the start of the study.

Soy isoflavones, lycopene from cooked tomatoes, soy isoflavones, green tea polyphenols and cruciferous vegetable sulphoranes also prevent prostate cancer.

Most men over age 70 will have evidence of localized, indolent prostate cancer *in situ* at autopsy. Fortunately, it is usually very slow growing (indolent). Survival in localized disease without treatment is similar to age-matched controls. However, if the cancer begins to press on surrounding tissues, symptoms can arise such as urinary urgency, urinary hesitancy, urinary obstruction, terminal hematuria, nocturia, and pain in the pelvis or spine. Thrombo-embolism (clot in a vein) occurs in about 10% of cases. While early prostate cancer is relatively benign, once it is advanced and hormone-refractory it is likely to metastasize and median survival is only 6 to 12 months. Screening should begin by age 40 in high-risk patients, and by age 50 in others. A history of vasectomy is no longer considered a risk for prostate cancer. An annual digital rectal exam (DRE) by a physician can detect hard asymptomatic nodules in accessible areas of the gland.

PSA TESTS

- Prostate specific antigen (PSA) reflects the total amount of prostate tissue, and is a good screen for abnormal growth of the gland. Normal range is 0 - 4. The i deal range is below 2.5. Benign prostatic hypertrophy (BPH) will not put PSA above 4, but 35% of men with early prostate cancer will show normal range PSA values.
- PSA Velocity monitoring steps up testing to every 6 months if the PSA increases by a value of 1 or doubles within one year.
- When PSA is in the range of 4 to 10 check *free PSA* or unbound antigen. If over 25% is in the free form, the chances of cancer are only 5 - 8%. When free PSA is under 10% there is a 56% chance there is cancer.
- Proenzyme PSA (pPSA) is more sensitive than free PSA. If the percentage of pPSA exceeds the PSA level it is a strong indicator of cancer.
- After effective treatment of prostate cancer the PSA will often drop into the normal range. Further monitoring should employ the 'ultra-sensitive PSA' test.

LAB TESTS

- standard work-up with CBC, Chem panel and U/A
- alkaline phosphatase detects bone mets
- prostatic acid phosphatase
- PSMA
- p-27 marker for aggressiveness, risk of mets and mortality
- IGF-1 is 4 times stronger stimulator of PCa than testosterone!
- Insulin, prolactin, testosterone and DHEA hormones
- blood clotting factors

IMAGING & SCANS

- trans-rectal prostatic ultrasound locates lesions and measures the volume of the gland, useful to calculate the "PSA density". Prostate cancer cells make more PSA than normal prostate cells, so high output from a small gland confirms the presence of cancer.
- needle biopsy
- endorectal MRI to rule out capsule penetration
- CXR, CT scan, bone scan and prostascint scans to rule out mets to bone, lymph and lung
- PET scans

GLEASON SCORE

Scores the degree of abnormality in the biopsied cells, with high numbers indicating a worse prognosis:

    2 to 4   = well differentiated
    5 to 7   = moderately differentiated
    8 to 10 = poorly differentiated

Score of 7 gives a 48% 5 year survival
Score of 8 gives a 25% 5 year survival

The Partin tables are a nomogram which uses the Gleason score, PSA and clinical assessment to determine if patients are likely to benefit from surgery. The 3 variables are combined in a multinomial log-linear regression to give a percent predictive probability, with 95% confidence that the patient will progress to a given final pathological stage.

The patients at high risk for reoccurrence after primary therapy:

- Gleason score over 8. However, prognosis is better if the PSA is still under 10.
- PSA reoccurs within 2 years of primary therapy
- PSA doubling in less than 6 months with a slope >0.15
- Initial PSA greater than 20
- Reoccurrence in the axial skeleton shows a median survival of 53 months, while reoccurrence in the appendicular skeleton has a median survival of 29 months.
- Advanced metastatic prostate cancers can over-express EZH2 messenger RNA and EZH2 protein, which mediates cell proliferation, cellular memory, and transcriptional repression. Higher levels of this biomarker in tissue samples indicates an aggressive and advanced cancer.

STAGING

The Jewett system designates stages A & B as local disease, C is invasive, and D is widespread. The TNM system is also used.

Stage A or T1: clinically undetectable by DRE or imaging, found at surgery.
Stage A1 or T1a: well-differentiated focal tumor.
Stage A2 or T1b: moderately or poorly differentiated tumor, may have multiple foci.
Stage T1c: elevated PSA, needle biopsy positive.
Stage B or T2: tumor confined to prostate, detectable by palpation or imaging.
Stage B0 or T2a: non-palpable, detected by PSA, involves less than ½ of one lobe of the gland
Stage B1 or T2b: single nodule in over ½ of one lobe.
Stage B2 or T2c: more extensive tumor in one or both lobes.
Stage C or T3: disease extends through the prostate capsule and may involve the seminal vesicles.
Stage C1 or T3a: clinical unilateral extra-capsular extension
Stage T3b: bilateral extra-capsular extension
Stage T3c: extends to the seminal vesicles
Stage C2: extension causing bladder outlet or urethral obstruction
Stage D or T4: metastatic beyond the seminal vesicles.
Stage D0: persistently elevated serum acid phosphatase
Stage D1: invades regional lymph nodes
Stage T4a: involves bladder neck, external sphincter or rectum
Stage D2: distant lymph nodes positive , mets to bone or visceral organs
Stage T4b: fixed to pelvic wall or involving levator muscles
Stage D3: relapse of prostate cancer after adequate endocrine therapy

MEDICAL TREATMENT OF PROSTATE CANCER

SURGERY

SYSTEMATIC SEXTANT BIOPSY - provides a Gleason grade. In localized prostate disease it can be used to predict risk of lymphatic spread by calculating it in a formula called the "Hamburg algorithm".

PROSTATECTOMY - radical surgery has the potential to cure as long as the disease is within the gland capsule. Preferred for younger men in stage A or B. Radical prostatectomy causes urinary incontinence in 54% of patients and erectile difficulties in 75% of cases. Early complications include rectal injury, thrombo-embolism, heart attacks, sepsis, anastomotic urinary leakage; mortality rate is 1 - 2%. Late complications include impotence, incontinence and cancer relapse. Impotence rates used to be about 95%. Recent trends to nerve-sparing surgery have reduced post-op impotence problems to about 60% for the short term - but still up to 75% long term.

LYMPHADENECTOMY - surgical resection of lymph nodes.

ORCHIECTOMY - surgical castration or resection of the testes to remove testosterone hormone stimulation in stage D prostate cancer.

CRYOSURGERY - freezing off tissue layers is technically demanding, but equals or exceeds other surgical and radiotherapy techniques in efficacy, and has a relatively low rate of complications.

RADIATION

EXTERNAL BEAM - using conventional X-ray and gamma ray sources; 3-D conformational style using leaflets to limit the treatment area; proton beams.

SEED IMPLANTS - moderate dosage over a long duration.

BRACHYTHERAPY - pellets of radioactive material such as Cesium, passed through the gland in a catheter, very high dose but short duration. Used in all stages from A to palliation in late D. It treats regionally. Radiotherapy may provoke less incontinence and impotence than surgery, but will make later surgery more difficult, and has a lower cure rate than surgery alone. The perineum is highly innervated, and is very reactive to both surgery and radiation. Radiotherapy complications can include radio-enteritis, radio-cystitis, impotence in 75%, urinary incontinence in 38%. Fecal incontinence, loose stools and stool leakage occur after radiotherapy at rates 3.6 times higher than seen from radical prostatectomy surgery.

HORMONE BLOCKADE

Hormone blockade starves the cancer of growth promoting factors on a systemic or body-wide basis. It is useful in advanced disease or as an alternative to radiation and surgery. However, resistance commonly occurs in 5 to 6 years, and there can be increased risk of death from infections and cardiovascular diseases. Other complications may include impotence, reduced libido, breast enlargement, muscle wasting, muscular weakness, acceleration of osteoporotic bone loss, and hot flashes. Note that drugs like Flutamide which specifically block testosterone receptors give no survival benefit, and cause depression, diarrhea and dementia.

Conventional wisdom says testosterone must be eradicated - by chemical or surgical castration. However, prostate cancer occurs at a time in a man's life when testosterone and progesterone production has sharply declined - and estradiol has risen. Remember testosterone and progesterone are estradiol antagonists, are far weaker carcinogens than estradiol, and stimulate p53 gene activity. Prostate cancer is also linked to exposure to estrogenic xenobiotics. The prostate gland has the same embryonic origin as endometrial tissue lining the womb - and endometrial cancer is clearly estrogen dependent. Estrogen stimulates the Bcl-2 oncogene, linked to prostate cancer as well as breast and endometrial cancers.

- Luteinizing hormone releasing-hormone analogues: Lupron, Zoladex. Lupron can cause hot flashes, reduce bone mineral density, raise triglycerides, and increase bad LDL cholesterol - but the adjunct use of soy ipriflavones counteracts these effects.
- Anti-androgens: Megace, Casodex, Eulixen
- Aromatase inhibitors: Arimidex
- Proscar
- Tamoxifen

Recent studies show hot flashes from prostate cancer therapy may respond well to acupuncture treatment twice a week, and also the newer anti-depressant drugs of the SSRI type (selective serotonin re-uptake inhibitors).

NATUROPATHIC TREATMENT OPTIONS IN PROSTATE CANCER

EXPECTANCY - watchful waiting is often appropriate in early prostate cancer as it is can be very slow-growing (indolent), there is uncertainty about the efficacy of many treatments, radical surgery and radiation frequently cause harsh side-effects, and the disease often occurs at an age where there are competing threats to mortality such as heart disease. Candidates for waiting with expectancy have:

- total sum Gleason score under 4
- diploid chromosomes = in normal pairs
- slow PSA rise (velocity) = under 1 ng/ml increase per year
- a life expectancy shorter than the natural course of prostate cancer - they are likely to die of something else first.

DIETETICS - diet may not cure the disease, but it heals the patient.

- Avoid red meat, fried foods, dairy, alcohol and sugar. Avoiding red meat, and using only low-fat white meats, low-fat dairy and emphasizing fish, fruit and vegetables will modulate and stabilize PSA, especially if weight loss is achieved.
- Saturated fat promotes metastases to bones.
- Trans-fatty acids as found in hydrogenated fats, margarine and shortening promote the formation of catechol estrogen-3, 4-quinone from estradiol and estrone, which destroys DNA purine bases.
- Omega-3 fatty acids from fish and nuts protect from these toxic estrogens. Also involved in these reactions are sulphur-containing amino acids, which we can get from eating beans, garlic, onions and leeks.
- Control insulin levels, as with the Schwarzbein Principle diet or the Matsen glycemic index diet. See: Basic Cancer Therapy Diet p.86 and Cancer Prevention Strategies p.202.

NATURAL PROGESTERONE - naturopathic doctors like to use normal physiological doses of natural forms of hormones only when they are proven to be deficient, as by saliva tests. Progesterone raises energy by stimulating anabolic metabolism, inhibits 5-alpha reductase conversion of testosterone into the more growth stimulating dihydotestosterone, and most importantly of all, antagonizes estrogens. We try to give 1 to 2 mg. per day as 1/8th tsp of a transdermal cream applied to the crook of the arm.

SAW PALMETTO - this herb is fine for slowing benign enlargement of the gland. However, it does not appear to have any significant role to play in treating prostate cancer. Do not mix with hormone blockade therapies.

DIM & I3C - diindolylmethane is activated indole-3-carbinol, which converts hormones like estrogen, progesterone and testosterone into less aggressive, less growth stimulating forms. It also induces arrest at G1 of the cell cycle, inducing apoptosis genes. I have seen it reduce PSA scores reliably.

FLAXSEED - mice bred to develop prostate cancer who were fed diets rich in flaxseeds (5% of their food intake) had half the number of tumors, and the tumors were far less aggressive and had a higher rate of apoptosis. The lignans in flax inhibit the development and the growth of prostate tumors. The lignans bind hormones and xenobiotics in the stool and increase sex hormone binding globulins in the blood. I have taken it for several years to prevent development of hormone dependent cancer.

SOY - soy foods are the most important dietary protectant from prostate cancer risk. Soy is rich in genestein, an isoflavone which inhibits growth of prostate cancer. Genestein competitively inhibits hormones at receptors, increases sex hormone blocking gonadotrophin, reduces growth signaling by tyrosine protein kinases, and is anti-angiogenic. Protein as found in soy foods helps maintain metabolic balance and immune competence.

MELATONIN - this pineal gland hormone down-regulates 5-lipoxygenase gene expression, prevents DNA oxidation, blocks the mitogenic effects of prostate cancer promoting hormones and growth factors, and reverses LHRH resistance. It will prolong life in late stage palliative care.

CURCUMIN - blocks formation of inflammatory cytokines PGE2 and HETE; significantly inhibits proliferation of prostate cancer cells; inhibits volume and number of prostate tumors by inhibition of angiogenesis and induction of apoptosis; may prevent progression of prostate cancer to a hormone refractory (resistant) state. LOX 5-HETE eicosanoid from arachidonic acid is as strong a growth stimulator for prostate cells as testosterone.

BOSWELLIA - inhibits tumor growth by inhibition of 5-lipoxygenase, DNA synthesis, and topoisomerases I & II.

VITAMIN D - slows the rise of PSA, inhibits cell cycle progression and may induce apoptosis. Inhibits IGF-1 which is a very strong growth stimulator for prostate cancer cells, even *more stimulating than testosterone*! Take as activated vitamin D3. Get sun on your skin in moderation. Use shade and mild aloe sunscreens to prevent sunburn.

VITAMIN E - VES inhibits prostate cancer cell growth and induces apoptosis in a dose-dependent manner. It significantly reduces mortality from prostate cancer. Vitamin E is synergistic with lycopene and selenium.

OLIVE OIL - the best inhibitor of PGE2 synthesis by prostate cancer cells, which are able to convert AA to PGE2 at a rate 10 times higher than benign prostatic hypertrophy (BPH) cells. Inhibition of 5-HETE induces massive apoptosis in prostate cancer cells.

QUERCITIN - inhibits 5-HETE to reduce inflammation, as does curcumin and melatonin. Inhibits aromatase to remove estrogenic stimulation.

GREEN TEA EGCG - inhibits growth of prostate cancer by a variety of mechanisms including inhibition of 5-alpha reductase, anti-angiogenesis, arrest of cell cycle at G2-M and by inducing apoptosis.

ZINC - the prostate collects high concentrations of zinc. Zinc is useful for prevention and treatment of benign prostate enlargement (BPH).   Zinc inhibits prostate cancer growth by increasing activity in gene p21, increasing apoptosis, inhibiting 5-alpha reductase, and binding prolactin and dihydrotestosterone.

RUTIN - polyphenols in red wine induce apoptosis in prostate cancer cells. The inhibition of tumor growth was highest from the rutin, gallic acid and tannic acid, and less from the quercitin and morin polyphenols.

MILK THISTLE - slows prostate cancer growth, inhibits EGF.

Other natural treatments - stinging nettles, vitamin C, vitamin K, selenium, modified citrus pectin, GLA oils, garlic.

Note that DHEA supplements must be avoided as they boost IGF-1 and sex hormones. Sterols and sterolins can increase DHEA levels and reduce cortisol levels. The IGF-1 production in the liver is increased by DHEA and also its biological activity rises due to induced changes in IGF-binding proteins. IGF stimulates growth of all prostate cells, with or without cancer

Chondroitin supplements used for arthritis may increase the spread of prostate cancer.

Chapter Twelve - INTEGRATIVE CARE OF COLORECTAL CANCER

EPIDEMIOLOGY

Colorectal carcinoma (CRC) is of course linked to the food passed through these organs. A high-fat, low fiber diet, alcohol and low intake of vitamin C, folate, calcium, selenium, flavones and indoles are all risk factors. 94% of cases are over 50 years old. Risk goes up the more red meat you eat, and down with eating more vegetables, including tomatoes. Sedentary habits put you at risk. A history of breast or endometrial cancer increase risk. People with a history of inflammatory bowel diseases such as Crohn's regional enteritis or ulcerative colitis (UC) have increased risk of CRC. Central adiposity (fat around the waist and viscera of the belly) is a risk factor, and is associated with insulin resistance, high insulin and IGF growth factors, especially IGF-2 overexpression.

Most colorectal cancers start as benign polyps in the colon. Familial polyposis syndrome puts some people at higher risk. The stem cells in the colonic crypt produce enterocytes which mature, migrate to the top of the crypt and are shed into the lumen of the colon. Polyps are hyperplastic growths which can become inflamed and degenerate into neoplastic adenomas, followed by invasion through the crypt walls, and metastasis. Prevent cancerous conversion by folate, calcium D-glucarate, fibre, probiotic and antioxidant supplementation.

Once CRC has occurred, there is a 20% chance another will occur within 5 years.

SYMPTOMS & SCREENING

- Patients may have vague abdominal pains, sometimes mimicking peptic ulcers.
- There may be alteration in the bowel habit and tenesmus (urging but nothing will pass).
- There is often a low grade chronic but intermittent blood loss detectable by stool testing for occult blood.
- Carcinoembryonic antigen (CEA) may be elevated, in direct relation to the size and extent of the tumor. When high, the prognosis is poorer. CEA will also be elevated from alcoholic cirrhosis, ulcerative colitis, pancreatitis, and cancers of the breast, ovary, bladder and prostate.
- Colonoscopy is preferred to sigmoidoscopy, to detect adenomatous polyps and colonic carcinomas high up in the bowel.
- 3 to 5% of small polyps are carcinomas
- COX-2 inhibitors reduce polyp conversion to neoplasia.

TUBULAR ADENOMA

75% of neoplastic polyps are tubular adenomas.

Invasiveness varies with size:

- under 1 cm diameter = 1% chance of invasive tumor
- 1 to 2 cm diameter = 10% chance
- over 2 cm diameter = 45% chance

VILLOUS ADENOMA

The larger and less common polyp, occurring in the recto-sigmoid area, or on the right in the cecum or ascending colon. 30% are invasive cancers, and they metastasize freely. Frequently associated with bleeding and a protein-rich mucus secretion.

This leads to frank blood and mucus from the rectum, fatigue, and malnutrition. Blood tests may show low protein, low albumin and low potassium.

LEFT-SIDED CRC

62% of CRC is left-sided. *In situ* CRC develops in 1 to 2 years into annular lesions encircling the bowel. The infiltrated gut wall is flattened and may show mucosal ulceration. These produce characteristic "napkin-ring" constrictions, seen with X-rays taken with a barium contrast enema. The early warning signs are a change in bowel habit to diarrhea or constipation, and melena (blood in the stool).

RIGHT-SIDED CRC

38% of CRC is right-sided. These lesions tend to be clinically silent until quite large, as the cecum is spacious. Bulky, fungating, cauliflower-like tumor protrudes into the lumen. There may be weakness and malaise, anemia and weight loss.

METASTASIS

Any CRC can dissect the gut wall and invade by direct extension into adjacent tissues. Metastasis is via lymphatics and blood vessels to the regional lymph nodes, liver, lungs, bone, brain and the peritoneal serosal membrane.

FIVE YEAR SURVIVAL RATES

Colon:	localized	- 88%	spreading	- 58%
Rectal:	localized	- 80%	spreading	- 47%

MODIFIED DUKE'S CLASSIFICATION

A - limited to mucosa
B - invading deeper layers, 1 in 4 will be fatal
B1 - into muscle layer, nodes clear
B2 - through the entire gut wall, nodes clear
C - regional spread, more than ½ of cases will die from it
C1 - in gut wall and node positive
C2 - through the entire wall and node positive
D - distant metastatic spread

MEDICAL TREATMENT OF COLORECTAL CANCER

SURGERY

If under 3 cm. diameter (just over an inch), local resection to remove the tumor plus adjacent mesenteric lymph nodes can be curative.
Larger rectal lesions may result in a temporary colostomy, only 15% will have to have a permanent colostomy. Large or obstructive tumors may be debulked with radiation before surgery. Check CEA before surgery. 2% may die from the surgery.

RADIATION

Pre-operative radiotherapy at just 5 fractions in 1 week may do more than chemotherapy or post-operative radiotherapy. Post-op adjuvant radiation in about 28 fractions over 6 weeks can improve survival where the tumor has penetrated the gut wall, involves the regional lymph nodes, is within 15 cm. of the anal verge, or has invaded the small intestine, bladder, ovaries or uterus.Palliative radiation for inoperable tumors, for pain or excess bleeding gives 90% of cases relief within 6 weeks. Dukes stage B2 or C rectal cancers do better with radiation plus chemotherapy.
Patients with higher levels of p53 mutations are unresponsive to radiotherapy and have reduced survival.

CHEMOTHERAPY

The chemo drug of choice is 5-fluorouracil. Adjunctive chemo agents include levamisole or leucovorin (calcium folinic acid). Vitamins C & E synergize with 5-FU.
The response rate is poor at 20%. Adjuvant chemo does not help those with high frequency microsatellite instability in their tumor DNA. The nausea and diarrhea can be severe, and will benefit from L-glutamine supplementation. Myelosuppression is also a risk - the bone marrow is injured, so blood cells cannot be created.

Irinotecan is a topoisomerase inhibitor which inhibits cell division by inducing single strand DNA breaks. It can be useful with or after 5-FU with leucovorin rescue.

Oxaliplatin is a third generation platinum compound which cross-links DNA, inducing apoptosis. It is synergistic with 5-FU.

IMMUNOTHERAPY

CRC produces antigens recognizable by T-cells. Monoclonal antibodies are useful after surgery, and repair post-surgical immunosuppression. Edrecolomab is monoclonal Ig2A antibody to human CRC Ep-CAM antigen.

NATUROPATHIC TREATMENT OPTIONS IN COLORECTAL CANCER

Colorectal cancer is very much a consequence of the modern agricultural diet with high carbohydrates, low fiber, low calcium, and damaged fats. Traditional hunter-gatherer dietary ingredients such as nuts and oil seeds and fish help prevent CRC. As Dr. Diana Shwarzbein says, it is best if it could be hunted, fished, milked, picked or gathered.

FOLATE - folic acid or its salt folate are B vitamins highly protective against colorectal cancer. It methylates and silences DNA. Folate is very high in green leafy vegetables, such as salad greens.

PROTEIN - support protein status, with whey protein powder such as HMS 90, and L-glutamine.

FISH OILS - omega 3 oil dihexanoic acid (DHA) reduces polyps, especially larger ones, lowers risk of conversion to CRC. Eicosapentanoic acid (EPA) induces cAMP to re-differentiate CRC. Seal oil or cod liver oil may also be used.

VITAMIN D - Inhibits CRC cell proliferation by regulating DNA transcription in well-differentiated tumors expressing the cytoplasmic vitamin D receptor. Rx: 5000 I.U. 3 to 7 days a week. *Serum calcium must be monitored.* Cod liver oil is a good source of DHA, EPA, vitamin A and vitamin D.

CALCIUM - inhibits proliferation, increases differentiation in human colonic cells. Calcium carbonate is cheap, and is poorly absorbed above the colon; use 1,200 mg.

FIBER -
- Eat lots of dietary fiber as organic vegetables and fruits, and whole grains.
- Binds cytotoxic unconjugated bile acids, steroid hormones and xenobiotics.
- Provides media for good bacterial flora and fauna to produce short chain fatty acids, such as butyrates which strongly regulate the DNA.
- Lowers insulin levels.
- Lowers gut pH (increases acidity)

VITAMIN E - VES arrests CRC tumor cells in G1 phase, leading to apoptosis. It is associated with increased survival time in terminal CRC, combined with omega 3 oils.

QUERCITIN - inhibits EGF receptor kinase to induce apoptosis in CRC, inhibits expression of p21-ras mutations, inhibits growth by binding to ER-II receptors, etc.

CURCUMIN - highly chemopreventative in CRC. Induces heat shock protein HSP 70. Reduces inflammation.

GRAPESEED proanthocyanins with glutathione e.g. *Recancostat* improves survival in poly-metastatic CRC with some restoration of body weight and quality of life.

PSYCHOLOGY - physicians will find CRC patients are often poorly compliant and treatment resistant. They tend to internalize stress. Empower them with control. They need creativity, art and self-expression.

Other treatment options in CRC
- exercise
- regulation of insulin & IGF
- lycopenes and carotenes
- treat food allergies and sensitivities
- probiotics - restore the beneficial gut bacteria ecology
- calcium D-glucarate 1.5 gm to detox xenobiotics and hormones.
- melatonin
- folate
- selenium
- DIM - diindolylmethane
- ImmunoCal *HMS 90* whey protein isolate as a glutahione precursor. Combine it with grapeseed extract.

Chapter Thirteen - INTEGRATIVE CARE OF LUNG CANCER

EPIDEMIOLOGY

A very common cancer with high mortality. Regional and distant spread is common. More than half of cases will have widespread metastases at the time of first diagnosis and will not survive for a year. The most significant causative factor is tobacco smoking. 30 pack years of cigarettes increases risk 20 times over non-smokers. Risk for a non-smoking spouse of a smoker is up 30%. Risk falls back near normal about 10 years after quitting smoking. Tobacco also increases risk of leukemia, as well as cancer of the mouth, esophagus, stomach, pancreas, pharynx, larynx, kidney, ureter, bladder, and cervix. It increases risk of cardiovascular disease (CVD) such as heart attack and stroke, and of course causes chronic lung diseases (COPD) such as emphysema. See p.181 for tips to discontinue tobacco abuse.

Exposure to radon gas entering a home from the ground and rock below can more than double risk of lung cancer, even at levels well below the official guidelines. The effect is additive and synergistic with tobacco smoke. Other independent and additive risk factors include tuberculosis, arsenic, and radiation exposure.

Bronchogenic cancers arising from the bronchial endothelial lining constitute 90% of lung cancers - squamous cell, large cell, small cell, broncho-alveolar and adenocarcinoma.

SYMPTOMS

Cough, sputum, hemoptysis (coughing up blood), respiratory stridor (breathing with great effort), upper respiratory infections (URI).
Paraneoplastic manifestations include ACTH and HGH irregularities.

NON-SMALL CELL LUNG CANCER (NSCLC)

75% of lung cancers, 4 subtypes with clinically similar behaviour -squamous epidermoid, adenocarcinoma, large cell and undifferentiated.
Slow growing, no rapid impact on quality of life. Often diagnosed after 5 to 8 years of growth. Typically found as a space-occupying lesion on a routine chest X-ray or CT. The lesion may be directly biopsied, and sputum cytology, fiber optic bronchoscopy washings or brushings, aspiration of pleural effusions, biopsy of nodes or metastatic tumors can also provide a diagnosis. Proteomic analysis of protein expression and post-translational modifications reflects the biochemical pathology and assist in making a prognosis of node involvement and of mortality.

Non-small cell lung cancer has a low response rate to chemotherapy, but there is potential for surgical cure if it is found while still localized.

Overall 5 year survival is 15%. Significantly poorer survival and relapse-free survival is seen in tumors expressing the cell adhesion molecule CEA CAM1. Such cases warrant aggressive adjuvant treatment.

STAGING NSCLC PRIMARIES

TX – positive sputum or washings, no tumor

Tis – carcinoma in situ

T1 – tumor under 3 cm diameter

T2 – tumor 3 cm or more, or involving mainstem bronchus or visceral pleura, or subtotal atelectasis, or subtotal obstructive pneumonitis.

T3 – tumor invading the chest wall, diaphragm, mediastinal pleura, or atalectasis or obstructive pneumonitis of the entire lung.

T4 – tumor invading the mediastinum, esophagus, heart, great vessels of vertebral body. Malignant pleural effusion.

N0 – no regional lymph node metastases

N1 – in hilar or peribronchial ipsilateral nodes.

N2 – in mediastinal or subcarinal ipsilateral nodes

N3 – in any scalene or supraclavicular nodes or contralateral hilar or mediastinal nodes

M0 – no distant metastases

M1 – distant metastases

Occult:	TX	N0	M0
Stage 0 :	Tis	N0	M0
Stage I:	T1-2	N0	MO
Stage II:	T1-2	N1	M0
Stage IIIA:	T3	N0-1	MO
	T1-3	N2	M0
Stage IIIB:	T4	N0-2	M0
Stage IV:	any T,	any N	M1

SURGERY FOR NSCLC

Stage I - 5 year survival is about 45%

Stage II - 5 year survival is 20 - 25%

Stage IIIA – can be treated surgically in some cases

Stage IIIB and IV – cannot be cured with surgery.

RADIATION FOR NSCLC

Radiation is sometimes given after surgery, or in late disease, but the lungs are very sensitive to radiation, and when they scar up they cannot move air. Radiotherapy actually increases early deaths about 21% in early NSCLC. Give high dose vitamin E, N-acetyl cysteine and grapeseed extract to prevent harm.

Acute radiation pneumonitis may follow 1 to 6 months after therapy., with bloody cough, chest pain and breathing distress.

Medication is usually prednisone, azathioprine or cyclosporine A.

Taxol is radio-sensitizing for lung tissue, as are taxanes in yew bark tea.

CHEMOTHERAPY FOR NSCLC

NSCLC – Cisplatin, carboplatin, mitomycin, vinblastine, ifosfamide, gemcitabine, and paclitaxel.

The new drug Iressa is an epidermal growth factor inhibitor showing some efficacy, but is linked to deaths from interstitial pneumonia.

SMALL CELL LUNG CANCER (SCLC)

Small or oat cell carcinoma (SCLC) accounts for about 25% of lung cancers. It follows a very rapid clinical course, with survival of only
1 to 2 months in extensive disease. Survival is only 4 to 5 months in limited stage disease, which is defined as tumor in one hemithorax and regional lymph nodes, including ipsilateral (same-side) supraclavicular adenopathy (swollen nodes above the collarbone) and pleural effusion.

CHEMOTHERAPY FOR SCLC

- A platinum drug is usually combined with a second chemo drug i.e. cisplatin + etoposide from podophyllotoxin is often the treatment of choice.
- Variations include the less toxic carboplatin, plus doxorubicin, cyclophosphamide, gemcitabine or taxol (as docetaxel or paclitaxel)
- Limited stage disease will respond 80-90% of the time, with 12 to 18 months until reoccurrence.
- Extensive stage disease will respond 60-80% of the time with 7 to 10 months until reoccurrence. Chemotherapy for metastatic NSCLC is always palliative.
- In mesothelioma the standard of care is cisplatin with pemetrexed. Pemetrexed is a multitarget (3 enzymes) anti-folate which inhibits DNA synthesis. This drug combination has a 41% response rate - average survival is 12 months.
- Monoclonal antibodies targeting the epidermal growth factor receptor (EGFR) can cause regression of adenocarcinoma and squamous cell carcinoma of the lung, with symptomatic improvement.

NATUROPATHIC TREATMENT OPTIONS IN LUNG CANCER

SMOKING CESSATION - to quit smoking take L-glutamine or Thorne research Sulfonil to reduce cravings.   Take grapeseed extract OPC's and N-acetyl-cysteine to neutralize toxins. Homeopathic *Tabacum* 6C is detoxifying, and may be included in the calming tincture of oatstraw *Avena sativa*. Be nice to yourself.

I like to "staple" the ear acupuncture points Shenmen, Liver and Lung, or for the weaker patient I may apply silver magrain pellets, which do not break the skin. TCM acupuncture points include LI-4, LI-20, ST-36, LV-3, PC-6, and the great trilogy at the radial wrist: LU-7, extra point Tim Mee, and a delicate puncture of "Dr. Cheung's Secret Point" which enters above LI-5 and is directed down to the Lung meridian to LU-9 at the wrist crease.

MELATONIN - stabilizes cases with no liver mets and not more than one brain met. Significantly increases survival and time until progression.   Tumor response rate and one year survival doubles by combining melatonin with chemotherapy.

N-ACETYL-CYSTEINE - NAC is mucolytic and a lung protectant antioxidant.

VITAMIN E - lung protectant antioxidant.

FEI LIU PING - for primary bronchogenic cancer.

LIU WEI DI HUANG WAN - for deficient lung yin, as in small cell cancer; if the kidney yang is weak substitute Ba Wei Di Huang Wan. Enhances chemotherapy outcomes.

ASTRAGALUS - a TCM chi tonic herb, often found in liquid extracts with ginseng, significantly enhances survival with small cell lung cancer.

Other care options in lung cancer -
- Vitamin C
- Iscador injectable mistletoe
- Can Z (Ping Xiao Pian) or Internal Dissolution Pills
- Photodynamic therapy with ionized oxygen

Chapter Fourteen - INTEGRATIVE CARE OF OVARIAN CANCER

EPIDEMIOLOGY

The cause is unknown, but ovarian cancer is associated with cancers of the breast, colon, or uterus; BRAC1, BRAC2, or p53 gene over-expression; obesity, hypertension, diabetes; nulliparity or low parity, infertility, ovarian cysts, ovulatory drugs; exposure to talcum powder in the perineal area, antihistamines, antidepressant drugs, benzodiazepine tranquilizers, hair dyes; sedentary lifestyle, and lack of sunlight. 5 to 10% of cases are familial. Prolonged unopposed estrogen replacement therapy (without progesterone) increases risk 80% after 10 to 19 years of use.   Diets high in saturated fat, eggs, milk and cholesterol raise risk, while legumes and vegetables are protective. Risk is reduced after taking oral contraceptives more than 5 years, tubal ligation, breast feeding, pregnancy and early menopause. Aspirin 3 times per week reduces risk 40%, possibly by cycloxygenase inhibition. Vitamin E and C at low doses reduce risk by 60%.

Age at onset is typically 55 to 59.   Symptoms are non-specific, and include vague pelvic or abdomenal discomfort, abdomenal swelling, indigestion, urinary frequency, irregular menses, abnormal vaginal bleeding, blood clots, ascites, diarrhea, constipation, appetite changes, weight loss, shortness of breath. Palpable abdominal masses under 8 cm. in premenopausal women are usually benign. If a lumpy mass persists over 2 months, appears to grow, or develops after menopause, it should be investigated as ovarian cancer. Metastasis into the abdomenal cavity is common even with small tumors, so most ovarian cancers are at an advanced stage when diagnosed. There is a 75% reoccurrence rate, and recurrent tumors tend to be very drug-resistant.   Prognosis is improved when the tumor is debulked before chemo, often by surgery.

HISTOLOGICAL TYPES

- 80 to 90% of ovarian cancers are epithelial adenocarcinomas; clear cell variant has the poorest prognosis
- germ cell tumors account for less than 5%, arise in teens to early 20's, aggressive but amenable to chemotherapy
- stromal tumors - rare
- low malignant potential tumors - rare indolent low-grade serous carcinomas have a 5 year survival rate of over 60%, but are unresponsive to chemotherapy. Generally these are fatal by about 10 years. Most of these tumors have mutations in BRAF or KRAS genes associated with kinase signalling cascades.

STAGING

Stage I – 15% of cases, disease is limited to ovaries

Stage II – 15% of cases, there is extension of disease into pelvic tissues

Stage III – 65% of cases, peritoneal implants, which spread by local
extension into the omentum, diaphragm & liver

Stage IV – 5%, distant metastases

SCREENING & DIAGNOSIS

Pelvic exam may be followed by abdomenal or transvaginal ultrasound. CT or PET scans are sometimes done. Tumor markers include CA-125, AFP, HCG or LPA (lysophosphatidic acid). The risk of malignancy index (RMI) is calculated as a product of CA-125 level, an ultrasound score, and a score for the patient's menopausal status.

SURGERY

Debulking, oophorectomy or total abdomenal hysterectomy (TAH). After a second-look laparoscopy, check CBC, chemscreen and CA-125 quarterly for at least 2 years.

RADIATION

External beam sources or local radioactive phosphorus. Seldom used due to complications like GI enteritis, liver function changes, pulmonary fibrosis, and loss of hematogenous marrow. Can be considered for palliation of metastatic disease.

CHEMOTHERAPY

Commonly used agents are cisplatin, taxol, carboplatin, adriamycin, cyclophosphamide, and topetecan. Liposomal doxorubicin (Adriamycin) is also used. 2/3 relapse within 2 years of primary therapy. Cancers which relapse within 6 months are generally unresponsive to further chemotherapy. I.V. cisplatin is sometimes augmented with intraperitoneal cisplatin, which penetrates 1 - 2 mm or 6 - 8 cell layers. A new microtubule inhibitor Epotilone (EPO906) is better tolerated than platinum and taxol, and gives some responses in phase II trials with advanced refractory ovarian cancer.

HORMONAL THERAPY

Palliative last resort for patients who have failed cytotoxic chemotherapy, response rates are only 4 -15%. Anti-estrogens, anti-androgens, gonadal releasing hormone (GNRH) analogues.

IMMUNOTHERAPIES

IL-2, IP LAK cells, interferon, BCG, monoclonal antibodies.

NATUROPATHIC TREATMENT OPTIONS IN OVARIAN CANCER

This is a cancer usually diagnosed late after it has become old, cranky and widespread. This is a time to be aggressive with mistletoe injections and other immune therapies, morning and lunchtime.

MELATONIN - enhances IL-2 and chemotherapy responses. Reduces chemo toxicity. Improves quality of life and control in cases where no standard treatment is available.

SELENIUM - as selenite it is cytotoxic to ovarian cancer cells. Improves taxol and Adriamycin responses.

GLUTHIONE - reduces cisplatin neurotoxicity, improves chemo responses. Use N-acetyl cysteine or *HMS 90* whey extract.

QUERCITIN - dose-dependent inhibition of OC, down-regulates OC cell signal transduction, binds to type II estrogen receptors, aromatase inhibitor, inhibits high aerobic glycolysis, arrests OC cells in G0-G1 phase, inhibits development of heat shock proteins. Synergistic with both cisplatin and genestein.

SOY - inhibits hormone responsive tumors; enhances actions of chemo drugs, radiation, and quercitin; protease inhibitors block OC cell urokinase, inhibiting invasiveness. Soy isoflavones block IL-6 production and promote transforming growth factor beta (TGFb) which reduces ovarian cancer cell proliferation and viability by an estrogen dependent pathway. Protein supports metabolism and repair.

GREEN TEA EGCG - enhances Adriamycin uptake by OC cells, improving chemo response while inhibiting metastases.

CURCUMIN - dose-dependent toxicity to OC cells. Induces apoptosis.

MUSHROOM POLYSACCHARIDES - shitake lentinan corrects OC resistance to cisplatin or 5-FU. Coriolus PSK increases IL-2 by 2.5 fold, and also augments cisplatin therapy.

MILK THISTLE - dose-dependent inhibition of OC; potentiates cisplatin and Adriamycin responses.

GINSENG - dose-dependent inhibition of growth of OC cells by RH2 ginsenosides. Enhances response to cisplatin. Careseng ginsenoside preparations are given orally and intravenously.

VITAMIN A - vitamin A and retinoic acids induce differentiation, apoptosis and cell proliferation

VITAMIN D - synergistic with vitamin A. Many ovarian tumors are rich in vitamin D receptors, and OC is more common in areas with less sunlight.

DIM - diindolylmethane or indole-3-carbinol convert any stray hormones into mild forms which cannot stimulate tumor growth.

MISTLETOE - *Iscador* injectable mistletoe lectins are a vital biological response modifier (BRM).

Other natural supports to consider -
- Omega 3 fats
- CLA - conjugated linoleic acid
- N-acetyl cysteine
- vitamin E succinate
- bromelain
- gingko biloba
- graviola
- flaxseed

Chapter 15 - CARE OF UTERINE, CERVICAL & VULVAR CANCERS

CERVICAL CANCER

The widespread use of the Pap smear has reduced the death rate in North America from cancer of the cervix of the uterus. This valuable screening test was developed by Dr. George Papanicolaou in the 1930's. Rates can only fall so far, however, as this disease behaves as if it is sexually transmitted. Sexual behaviour remains as popular, and as impulsive and reckless as ever. The causative factor appears to be the human papilloma virus (HPV) which is also responsible for genital warts. There is a strong association with smoking tobacco, as the cervical mucus can secrete concentrates of cigarette carcinogens 10 to 20 times higher than seen in the blood. Risk from HPV rises sharply in smokers. Birth control pills in a person with folate deficiency is a risk.

Warning signs include abnormal bleeding - which may only be on contact, foul or bloody discharge, ulceration, pain in the back and pelvis, and weight loss. A Pap smear of grade IV is severe dysplasia, strongly suspicious for carcinoma in situ. Pre-invasive stages are slow-growing and usually asymptomatic. A Pap grade of V is invasive squamous cell carcinoma. 95% of biopsies will have human papilloma virus. Polyps on the cervix are rarely (1%) cancerous.

Allopathic treatment may follow a Pap test or biopsy guided by colposcopy. The conal biopsy technique removes localized cancer, and the cervical stump remains satisfactory for childbearing. Invasive cancer requires more radical surgery. Early treatment by surgery can be curative. However, it is resistant to cure once it has spread.

Radiation may be by implants, brachytherapy or external beam. The adjacent vagina, bladder and bowels are susceptible to inflammation and fibrosis from radiotherapy.

UTERINE CANCER

Often adenocarcinoma of the glandular epithelium of the corpus uteri – the endometrium. It is linked to exposure to unopposed estrogen. Early onset and late end of menses is a risk, as is obesity, polycystic ovary syndrome, birth control pills, hypertension and diabetes. Progesterone is protective, and can be used to reverse simple hyperplasia without atypia.

Early warning signs include spotting of blood between menses (metrorrhagia), any post-menopausal vaginal bleeding, colicky abdomenal pains, backache, leg edema, weight loss, and there can be a cough with bloody phlegm (hemoptysis).

VULVAR CANCER

Associated with human pappiloma virus HPV and smoking. Survival rates are good if the tumor is under 4.0 cm. and there is no nodal involvement.

NATUROPATHIC CARE OF CERVICAL CANCER

VITAMIN A - Vitamin A palmitate and beta carotene in very high doses strongly re-differentiate these cancers. Carotenes may be given to 200,000 units daily, and vitamin A at 50,000 I.U. or more daily, under close supervision by a physician.

FOLIC ACID - 5 to 10 milligrams daily can reverse early cervical dysplasia, and reduces carcinogenesis risk from human papilloma virus HPV types 16 & 18.

STEROLS & STEROLINS - can eradicate HPV in about 50% of cases.
I use Vitazan Sterol Complex with beta-sitosterols.

ESCHAROTICS – "Vaginal depletion packs" made by Eclectic Institute are professional naturopathic escharotics which can cure squamous cell carcinoma in situ. Active principles are vitamin A, oil of *bitter orange*, tea tree oil *Melaleuca cajeputi*, *Thuja occidentalis*, *Hydrastis*, *Phytolacca*, and magnesium salts. Dr. Tori Hudson, N.D. adds zinc chloride and *Sanguinaria*. The cervix may be cleaned with hydrogen peroxide and pre-treated with proteolytic enzymes before using the Vag-Pack paste. Repeat the Pap smear 3 months after treatment. Clinical studies have demonstrated a very high rate of remission.

Dr. John Bastyr, ND used an escharotic of 1 part saturated zinc chloride (ZnCl) to 3 parts tincture of *Sanguinaria*. The cervix is prepared with bromelain or chymotrypsin enzymes, rinsed with *Calendula* succus (marigold juice), painted with escharotic, including the endocervical canal, then rinsed with *Calendula* succus after the abnormal tissue has blanched (turned white).

PSYCHOLOGY - Dr. Christiane Northrup, M.D., author of *Women's Bodies, Women's Wisdom* suggests that low self-esteem, religious shame about sexuality, and passive or pessimistic reactions to stress can set the stage for more severe disease.

INDOLE-3-CARBINOL - Dr. Maria Bell, M.D. an oncologist at the University of South Dakota Medical Center has reported dramatic results with indole-3-carbinol (I3C), seeing in 12 weeks complete regression of stage 2 and 3 cervical cancer in 4 of 8 women dosed at 200 mg. daily, and 4 of 9 dosed at 400 mg daily. Those receiving placebo had no improvement.

FLAXSEED - reduces hormone stimulation.

Other options in cervical cancer - vitamin B6 - 150 mg.,
vitamin B12 - 1 mg., vitamin C - 1 gram, vitamin E - 400 I.U.,
zinc - 30 mg., and selenium - 400 mcg.

NATUROPATHIC CARE OF UTERINE CANCER

Hormone blockade:

- flaxseed
- quercitin
- diindolylmethane
- melatonin
- progesterone.

Consider also vitamin C, vitamin A, beta carotene and folic acid.

NATUROPATHIC CARE OF VULVAR CANCER

Survival rates are good if the tumor is under 4.0 cm and there is no nodal involvement.

Quit smoking

Adjuncts to strengthen the immune system and suppress the HPV:

- sterols & sterolins
- vitamin A
- ganoderma
- cat's claw

Chapter Sixteen - INTEGRATIVE CARE OF GASTROINTESTINAL
CANCERS - ESOPHAGUS, STOMACH, LIVER & PANCREAS

ESOPHAGUS

Risk factors for esophageal cancer include alcohol, tobacco, fungal toxins, pickled and preserved foods, and deficiencies of vitamins and minerals.   p63 gene expression is elevated early in squamous cell esophageal cancer.   This homologue of the tumor suppressor gene p53 probably plays a role in the development of this cancer.
Early detection is rare, lateral invasion and metastasis can occur very early, so most are diagnosed with disseminated disease. Metastasis is usually to the lungs, liver, bones and kidneys. First signs may be dysphagia, substernal pain, hoarse voice, coughing provoked by eating or drinking, hemorrhage and anemia.
Allopathic treatment begins with surgery, and may add adjunctive or palliative chemotherapy with 5-fluorouracil, cisplatin and mitomycin. Radiation is often used in palliation.
Naturopathic options include the TCM formulas Liu Wei Di Huang Wan and Yi Qi Yang Yin Tang.

STOMACH

Gastric cancer is usually adenocarcinoma. Risk factors include low intake of fruit and vegetables, high intake of dietary nitrites, pickled and preserved food; a history of pernicious anemia, atrophic gastritis, gastric ulcer, adenomas and family history of cancer of the stomach.
Early signs can include anorexia, early satiety, nausea, vomiting, epigastric discomfort mimicking peptic ulcer, anemia, and disseminated intravascular coagulation with consequent bruising and bleeding.
Surgery with radiation or chemotherapy - 5-fluorouracil, doxorubicin, methotrexate, cisplatin and etoposide. Survival rates are poor.
Naturopathic treatment options of special interest include:

- aloe vera juice
- curcumin
- quercitin
- cod liver oil
- vitamin C
- berberine
- Licorice root *Glycyrrhiza uralensis* extract induces apoptosis in gastric carcinoma cells, and strongly reduces inflammation.
- Treat for *Helicobacter pylori* ulcer causing bacteria, strongly associated with gastric cancers -mastic gum, Manuka honey, vitamin C, Thorne SF734, berberine.

TCM formulas of interest for stomach cancer:

- Pishen Fang
- Shen Xue Tang
- Juan Pi Yi Shen
- Shih Chuan Da Bu Wan
- Liu Wei Di Huang Wan
- Liu Wei Hua Jie Tang.
- Si Jun Zi Tang

LIVER

Hepatic cancer is associated with hepatitis B and C viruses, cirrhosis, alcohol, fungal aflatoxins, anabolic steroids, and xenobiotics. 90% are hepatocellular cancers. Early signs can include obstructive jaundice, hepatomegaly, splenomegaly, anorexia, fatigue, belly pain, ascites, weight loss and elevated liver enzymes. A drop in insulin-like growth factor 1 (IGF-1) correlates with development of hepatocellular carcinoma in cases of hepatitis C (HCV) cirrhosis. Serum alpha-fetoprotein (AFP) may also elevated, and is a useful marker during treatment. The favored chemotherapy is doxorubicin. Survival rates are very low.

A recent development is radiofrequency ablation of inoperable tumors under 4 cm. An umbrella-like needle array is put into the tumor, and radio waves heat the tissue to 80 - 100 + degrees celsius, causing coagulation. Percutaneous radiofrequency (PRF) ablation is as good as cryosurgery for initial success and complications, but is superior in preventing metastatic spread. PRF is also used for renal tumors.

Liver metastases are very common from a variety of other cancers, and are best treated with surgical resection and neoadjuvant chemotherapy. Cryotherapy can be performed on unresectable masses, with an average freezing time of 18 minutes.

NATUROPATHIC OPTIONS IN LIVER CANCER

- milk thistle
- Hoxsey formula
- ginseng or ginsenosides
- Internal Dissolution Pills
- *Ukrain*
- glutathione, alpha lipoic acid, N-acetyl cysteine, vitamin C, vitamin E, selenium
- grapeseed OPC's, green tea polyphenols and curcumin combination
- graviola leaf
- mistletoe lectin injections - *Iscador*

PANCREAS

Causative factors are unclear, but there is a correlation with exposure to PCBs (polychlorinated biphenyls) and organochlorines.

80% of cases have spread lymph nodes and 70% have liver mets at presentation. Treatment is poor. Survival is usually less than 2 years.

Early signs are often vague, such as back pain, depression, jaundice, weight loss, anorexia, hepatomegaly (swollen liver), dark urine and light colored stool.

MUC1 is a transmembrane mucin expressed by pancreatic cancer cells. The amount of IgG antibodies against MUC-1 circulating in the blood is a significant predictor of survival.

The favored chemo drug is 5-fluorouracil.

NATUROPATHIC CARE OF PANCREATIC CANCER
- Hoxsey formula
- Internal Dissolution Pills
- AntiCancerlin tablets
- mistletoe injections - *Iscador*
- *Careseng* ginseng
- soy genestein
- green tea polyphenol extract
- taheebo tea
- vitamin A
- selenium
- graviola leaf
- *Ukrain* (NSC-631570) is a semi-synthetic compound of an alkaloid from the botanical Chelidonium majus and thiophosphoric acid - which can nearly double the median survival of advanced unresectable pancreatic cancer patients, given alone or in combination with the chemo drug gemcitabine. So why take the gemcitabine? Use 5 to 20 mg. 2 to 3 times weekly.

Chapter Seventeen - INTEGRATIVE CARE OF SKIN CANCERS

Cancer of the skin is very common, and will happen to one in five North Americans. These are mostly preventable. 97% will be non-melanoma cancers with a high cure rate. Risk of extensive spread of non-melanoma skin cancers is high for basal cell carcinoma (BCC) on the nose, morpheaform BCC on the cheek, recurrent BCC in men, any skin cancer on the neck in men, location on the helix of the ear, eyelid or temple, and increasing size
pre-operatively.

BASAL CELL CARCINOMA

BCC arises in non-keratinized cells of the basal cell layer of the epidermis, grows slowly, rarely metastasizes, but can cause extensive local damage. The characteristic lesion is a 'rodent ulcer', a rolled indurated pearly edge with a depressed central area of necrosis; other lesions are nodular and spherical. Angiogenesis can produce characteristic telangiectasias, but there may be ischemic central necrosis. Neglected lesions of the head and neck can invade the subcutis and nerves and spread to the bones and lungs. Curettage and electrodessication, cryosurgery, laser or sharp excision may be used. Radiation is occasionally used in treatment, more often in palliation. Retinoids have some utility, as do platinum-based chemotherapy agents.

SQUAMOUS CELL CARCINOMA

SCC is a cancer of the keratinizing cells, with more potential for anaplasia, rapid growth, local invasion, and if untended, metastasis to regional lymph nodes and distant sites than BCC. Metastasis is more likely if the lesion is on a mucosal surface such as the lips or on an injury site such as a scar or ulcer. Ultraviolet from sunlight is the primary risk factor, but so are chemical carcinogens, inflammation, viral transformation, and mutations. The tumor may be very irregular, and often has a surface scale or crust. It may just look like a simple sore or inflamed spot that does not heal.

Surgery is common, and a variety of modalities are used, as for basal call carcinoma. Radiation can be an alternative to surgery for elderly patients if lesions are on the nose, lips, canthus and eyelid
Recombinant IL-2 improves survival in oral squamous cell carcinoma. IL-2 is synergistic with melatonin and plant sterols.

MALIGNANT MELANOMA

These dark lesions are less common, but much more dangerous. The melanocyte is of neural crest origin, and produces the brown-black pigment melanin. They occur in the skin, perianal area, rectum, vagina, upper digestive tract, and in the eye structures - choroid, iris and ciliary body. The incidence is rising world-wide. Damage from UV-B rays is a prominent causal factor. Dysplastic nevi are high risk for transformation to melanoma. However, ordinary moles do not need to be removed. The characteristic lesion is asymptomatic, has irregular borders, mixed pigmentation, with possible finger-like projections.

Treatment is based on the estimated tumor thickness (Breslow's) and level of invasion (Clark's) plus regional lymph node involvement. Using ultrasound and digital videomicroscopy, the thickness can be accurately assesed. Lesions over 1 millimeter thick necessitate sentinel lymph node sampling. Wide excision aroung the lesion is required. Local reoccurrence is associated with 70% mortality within 5 years.

Adjuvants include radiation, interferon alpha 2B, interleukin-2, cisplatin, vinblastine, DTIC, thiotepa, nitrosoureas, and taxanes. Recombinant vaccines and gene therapy are under investigation.

NATUROPATHIC CARE OF SKIN CANCERS

- Vitamin A, carotenoids, vitamin E and vitamin D are critical.
- Green tea reduces UV damage and inflammation, as do COX-2 inhibitors such as curcumin, grapeseed OPC's and omega 3 oils
- Escharotics as used by Hoxsey and Bastyr are useful alternatives, as is podophyllin resin.
- IL-2 is greatly enhanced by melatonin and plant sterols.
- Quercitin is particularly active against melanomas.
- Hoxsey tonic tincture with homeopathic *Carcinosum*.
- Vaccinations against smallpox (Vaccinia) and tuberculosis (BCG) are protective against melanoma. BCG can be injected right into melanoma nodules. This may give pause to the homeopaths to consider miasmatic and constitutional remedies.
- Antioxidants are particularly needed by the skin. Use a face cream of vitamin C, MSM, alpha lipoic acid, grapeseed extract and vitamin E to heal injury and prevent degeneration.
- *Iscador P* injectable mistletoe lectins from pine trees is a specific for skin cancers.

Chapter Eightteen - INTEGRATIVE CARE OF BRAIN CANCERS

Cancer of the central nervous system is becoming more prevalent in the elderly and in children. Unequivocal risk factors are exposure to ionizing radiation and immuno-suppression. Chlorine in water increases risk by the formation of trihalomethanes.

CNS tumors develop vasculature without the normal blood-brain barrier, allowing in toxins and proteins which cause edema. Thus even small lesions can compress adjacent vital structures within the closed vessel of the cranium. Brain tumors are not malignant in the sense that they may spread to other tissues, but high grade lesions are dangerous and spread within the brain. Gliomas are particularly invasive. Diffuse tumors are inoperable.

Symptoms arise from raised intracranial pressure, focal signs from edema and ischemia, and hydrocephalus from blocked CSF flow.
The traditional Chinese (TCM) doctors call this a damp condition of
the marrow with phlegm obstructing the channels.
- Headache is common, can be severe, persistent and is typically crescendo in presentation - relentlessly getting worse.
- Vomiting, especially on awakening, with or without nausea
- Neck and back pain at night or early in the day, usually worse laying down and improved when standing upright.
- Seizures are quite common with focal sensory and motor signs.
- Behavioural and personality changes.

MRI and stereotactic 3 dimensional guided needle biopsy techniques have improved diagnosis and treatment. Despite surgery and good medical care half of all cases will be fatal within one year. Only 20% are cured. Post-surgical radiation may improve survival time. Chemotherapy may include nitrosourea - carmustine (BCNU) and PCV: procarbazine, CCNU and vincristine. Meningiomas are estrogen dependent, so hormone therapies are used as adjuncts to surgery.

Corticosteroids are very useful as palliatives as they reduce the edema and swelling dramatically within 24 to 48 hours. This is less helpful in tumors that have metastasized to the brain from elsewhere, which are less edematous and tend to grow as firm spheres.

NATUROPATHIC CARE OF BRAIN CANCERS

Use all the fat-soluble therapies such as vitamin E, vitamin D, EPA, DHA, GLA, sterols and sterolins, and coenzyme Q10. The brain is fatty and needs a lot of anti-oxidant protection against lipid peroxidation. It uses more oxygen than any other tissue.

Grapeseed extract is excellent for the integrity of the blood-brain-barrier.

Boswellia reduces edema from brain tumors, as does curcumin. Use anti-inflammatory herbs aggressively.

Quercitin is particularly active against meningiomas, as it is an aromatase inhibitor, stopping local production of estrogen.

Use melatonin to extend life and regulate the pineal gland.

Consider Hoxsey tincture with nosode *Gliom* from Pascoe Pharmacy. To this I would suggest adding homeopathic *Conium*.

100% *GLA* oil dissolves gliomas on contact when placed in a surgically formed cavity within the tumors. GLA is found in borage and evening primrose oils.

The lectin agglutinin in Jimson weed *Datura stramonium* induces irreversible differentiation in astrocytic gliomas.

Detoxification from fat-soluble pesticides is warranted when history suggests high exposure. I use Pascoe Pharmacy homeopathic nosodes orally or transcutaneously, and supplement with Thorne Research Pesticide Removal formulation. The brown rice diet or other detox diets are prescribed. Foods to increase include beets, cilantro leaf, fish, walnuts, almonds, and of course, pure water.

Survival of brain cancer cases in China are reported to be increased by 4 to 5 times when traditional Chinese medicine (TCM) is integrated with the medical oncology care!

Ping Xiao Pian or Internal Dissolution Pills are useful to shrink tumors.

Can Ju Tan releives headache, vomiting and other effects of brain cancers.

The Chinese are using Fish Otolith Formula specifically for brain tumors. It's salty properties resolve blood stagnation and dissolve the masses.

The classic Zhen Gan Xi Feng Tang may be added to the program if the yang energy is agitated, creating wind.

Tianma Gouteng Tang also controls wind.

Xifeng Ruanjian Tang extinguishes wind and softens accumulations, to increase survival quite dramatically for brain tumors. The scorpions, centipedes and earthworms in the formula are strange to Westerners.

Bushen Huantan Tang is a simple all-plant formula which transforms phlegm, tonifies the kidney, and increases survival in brain cancer.

Wen Dan Tang transforms phlegm, rids dampness (edema) in the brain.

Liu Wei Di Huang Wan is a classic to restore kidney yin to control yang and uprushing wind. The patients will have thin, smooth, shiny red tongues. Restoring the kidney nourishes the root of all health - the connection with the vital essences and the ancestors - the DNA.

Yiguan Jian and Ji Ju Di Huang Wan are formulas which also tonify a yin deficiency. If the heat signs are more extreme use Longdan Xiegan Tang.

IMPORTANT NOTE: *Iscador* mistletoe extract and *Ukrain* injectables can cause swelling around the tumor, which will increase intra-cranial pressure.
Use *Iscador P* from pine trees for peripheral nerve cancers.

Cancer in the brain must be controlled quickly. Often the patient needs corticosteroids to bring down the swelling. Take any help the other professions can offer.

Chapter Nineteen - INTEGRATIVE CARE OF LEUKEMIA & LYMPHOMA

Cancer of the immune and blood cells tend to occur in the very young and the elderly. Fortunately the cure rates with allopathic oncology is reasonably good. Unfortunately the treatments are very harsh, and carry a significant risk of provoking other cancers. Naturopathic co-care or complementary medicine has a clear role in moderating the harm, and increasing the proportion who can be cured.

Acute leukemias are marked by rapid proliferation and disordered differentiation, with accumulation of large numbers of immature blast cells in the blood and bone marrow. Untreated, this can be fatal in a few weeks to a few months.

HODGKINS DISEASE

Hodgkin's (HD) cancer and inflammation of the lymphoid tissue appears to correlate with an altered immune response to the Epstein Barr virus of infectious mononucleosis, or surgery to lymphoid tissue such as tonsillectomy or appendectomy. Defects in cell-mediated immunity involving the T-cells are common, resulting in serious infectious complications.

Early signs include painless swollen lymph nodes, but they may become tender on consuming alcohol. There is a moderate to marked neutrophilic leukocytosis and thrombocytosis, elevated serum fibrinogen, zinc and copper, anemia, and pruritus (itchiness). The lungs, liver, spleen and bone marrow are often involved. Later signs may include anorexia, weight loss, fatigue and high fever with drenching sweats.

Diagnosis is often by needle biopsy of lymph nodes.

Radiation can be curative in 90% of stage I to IIA cases. Prognosis is poorer if bulky lesions advance into the mediastinal lymph nodes or are found below the diaphragm. In stage III and IV the treatment of choice is chemotherapy with ABVD - adriamycin, bleomycin, vinblastine, and dacarbazine; or MOPP- mechloroethamine, vincristine, prednisone and procarbazine; or BEACOPP combination.

NON-HODGKINS LYMPHOMA

NHL lymphomas may arise from many causes, including the viruses hepatitis-C, Herpes-6 and EBV, the bacteria *Helicobacter pylori*, and autoimmune disorders like rheumatoid arthritis. Diagnosis is usually by excisional biopsy. The condition is usually found when already well advanced by hematogenous spread. Treated with radiation, alkylating CHOP protocol chemotherapy, purine analogues, stem cell transplants, monoclonal antibodies, and BCL-2 antisense oligonucleotide therapy.

A new radioactive antibody compound Bexxar has shown high remission and response rates in low grade advanced stage NHL, with a single dose. Minimal side-effects are seen including moderately low blood counts and flu-like symptoms.

ACUTE LYMPHOBLASTIC LEUKEMIA

ALL is the most common pediatric leukemia. Causes include maternal deficiency in folate and maternal exposure to agricultural chemicals during pregnancy; paternal exposure in the workplace to paints, solvents, degreasers and chemical cleansers; childhood exposure to pesticides.

Acute leukemias present with symptoms associated with altered bone marrow production of red blood cells, white blood cells and platelets: fatigue, malaise, anorexia, bruising, low-grade fevers, anemia, and immunodeficiency.

ALL has a complete remission rate of 90% in children treated with the combination chemotherapy vincristine, prednisone and asparaginase. Remission maintainence with methotrexate and mercaptopurine gives 55 to 70% long term survival. Also used are melphalan, chlorambusil, topoisomerase inhibitors, anthracyclines and etoposide.

Adults with acute lymphocytic leukemia are treated with vincristine, prednisone, daunorubicin, methotrexate, cyclophosphamide, cytosine arabinoside, 6-thioguanine and 6-mercaptopurine, and possibly asparaginase. Response rates are 60 - 80% for adults, but the duration of remissions are considerably shorter, usually under two years.

A promising new agent being studied is the farnesyl transferase inhibitor (FTI) R115777, which has induced remissions or prolonged disease stabilization in acute leukemia. FTI's inhibit the oncogene *ras* pathway, a guanine nucleotide binding protein which functions upstream of one of the main signal transduction pathways controlling cell proliferation, morphology, stress response and survival. Ras is activated when bound to the plasma membrane, which is mediated by a post-translational modification known as farnesylation. The FTI may shift processing of Rho-B to an inactivated geranylated state, rather than the active farnesylated state. Myelosuppression is less with intermittent dosing than continuous infusions.

ACUTE MYELOCYTIC/MYELOMONOCYTIC LEUKEMIA

AML is the most common adult form of acute leukemia, and is the type most often seen to result from exposure to radiation or chemotherapy.

A viral like-illness with fatigue and malaise may be followed by pain in the long bones, ribs and sternum. Unlike ALL, AML has little peripheral lymph node involvement. There are occasionally skin lesions. Blast cells may cause leukostasis syndrome, and the blast crisis phase is often terminal. Watch the hygiene and immune competence of the oral and the peri-rectal areas. The leukemic cells secrete platelet-derived growth factors which cause the fibroblasts to turn the bone marrow spaces fibrotic.

AML is initially treated with cytarabine and daunorubicin, and commonly reinforced with autologous or allogenic bone marrow transplantation. Beware cell lysis syndrome with hyperuricemia and hyperuricuria.

CHRONIC MYELOCYTIC LEUKEMIA

CML is associated with an abnormal Philadelphia Ph chromosome, and is characterized by myeloid hyperplasia. Chronic leukemias tend to show up on routine blood tests as thrombocytosis, with elevated lactic acid dehydrogenase and elevated uric acid. CML may also exhibit hepatomegaly, and will usually involve splenomegaly. CML is treated with hydroxyurea and bisulfan, although they do not stop the progression of the disease. Remission periods in the chronic phase can be prolonged with alpha-interferon. Gleevec (Imatinib mesylate) is an expensive new selective inhibitor of tyrosine kinase BCR-ABL which can restore normal blood counts in interferon-resistant CML. Children may receive allogenic bone marrow transplantation; adults up to age 55 may find a donor, but mortality with transplants of these stem cells is about 20%.

CHRONIC LYMPHOCYTIC LEUKEMIA

The most common adult chronic leukemia, especially for men. There may be fatigue, shortness of breath or bleeding problems. The blood tests show lymphocytosis over 5,000 per cubic millimeter. The disease is generally indolent, but 3 to 10% are at risk of transformation into the aggressive lymphoma of Richter's syndrome, marked by night sweats, weight loss, abdomenal pain, and lymphadenopathy. CLL may be treated with chlorambucil and prednisone or flubarabine.

HAIRY CELL LEUKEMIA

HCL is a rare and indolent lymphocytic leukemia. HCL is treated with alpha-interferon or 2-chlorodeoxyadenosine.

MULTIPLE MYELOMA

This lymphoma is characterized by diffuse destruction of bone including lytic "punched-out" lesions in the cranium. Doxorubicin and thalidomide are used, but this combination has a high risk of causing deep vein thrombosis. Thalidomide alone will give a response in many relapsed cases, with some sedation, neuropathy and neutropenia as side-effects. Adding dexamethasone to the thalidomide doubles the response rate. A new regime uses vincristine, oral dexamethasone and pegylated liposomal doxorubicin. Doxorubicin plus Bortezomib proteasome inhibitor is very active against myeloma, even refractory cases.

NATUROPATHIC CARE OF LEUKEMIAS & LYMPHOMAS

IMPORTANT NOTE: Never use melatonin with these disseminated cancers, including multiple myeloma!

IMMUNE MODULATORS - such as plant sterols and sterolins.
Shih Chuan Da Bu Wan - which contains contains astragalus and ligusticum - is supportive in leukemias, as are the herbs cordyalis, iris versicolor, arctium lappa, eleutherococcus, ganoderma, cornus, ginseng, milletia, polygonatum and psoralea.

GINSENG - is synergistic with vitamin C against leukemia cells.

NOTOGINSENG - Panax pseudoginseng is anti-leukemic.

CAT'S CLAW - Una de gato alkaloids have shown in vitro activity against leukemia and lymphoma cells.

EPA OILS - in Hodgkin's disease, cytokine modulators like cod liver, fish or seal oil.

GOOSE BLOOD TABLETS - are used in lymphoma.

SAGE - Salvia miltiorrhiza is synergistic with lymphoma COP chemotherapy protocol.

VITAMIN D3 - at 16,000 I.U. three times weekly can put chronic myelomonocytic leukemia in remission.

CURCUMIN - synergizes with vitamin D, is directly cytotoxic, promotes apoptosis, and suppresses activation of transcription factors AP-1 and NF-kappa B in chronic myeloid leukemia cells

INDIRUBIN - from the botanicals *Idigofera tinctoria* or *Isatis tinctoria* as used in the TCM formula Dang Gui Long Hui Wan for CML. Indirubin inhibits cyclin dependent kinases and glycogen synthase kinase 3 involved in G1 cell cycle phase.

VITAMIN A - enhances bisulphan activity against CML, at 50,000 I.U. daily

ACUPUNCTURE - in acute leukemia Bl-18, BL- 23, GB-39.

QUERCITIN - inhibits leukemia cell proliferation. It binds growth factor receptors such as type II estrogen receptors in leukemia cells.
It arrests leukemia cells in G1-S interphase.

ATRA - All trans retinoic acid has survival benefit in APL.

VITAMIN E - can assist with oxidative stress when tumor load is high, such as during a blast crisis.

VITAMIN K2 - induces apoptosis in APL myelogenous leukemia.

VITAMIN B12 and folate - support normal blood cell formation. I give them as a high dose intramuscular injection on a weekly to monthly basis.

HOMEOPATHY - leukemia viruses may be defeated with the Heel brand homeopathics *Engystol* and also *Echinacea Compositum*. Use by injection twice weekly for 2 weeks and as oral tablets twice daily for 3 weeks. Homeopaths will take note that multiple myeloma and Hodgkin's lymphoma are based in a *Luetic* miasm.

MULTIPLE MYELOMA - use tetracycline, calcium, vitamin D, and soy imipriflavones to protect bones from lysis and thus reduce bone pain. Use anti-angiogenics!

Radiofrequencies from cellular mobile phones initially disrupt leukemia cells, but after 24 hours the surviving cells begin to grow aggressively. This Italian study used continuous exposure, and contradicts recent Australian animal studies showing no effect from these phones on cancer cells.

Chapter Twenty -   CANCER PREVENTION STRATEGIES

Bad things do happen to good people. No one should ever feel ashamed or blamed for developing cancer.   We are responsible for trying to do our best with the life we are given. There are winning strategies to reduce the risk and worry of cancer.

- Fats – As Udo Erasmus says, "fats can heal and fats can kill". Reducing dairy fat, margarine and shortening cuts out a lot of the carcinogenic trans fatty acids and lowers omega 6 oils. Reducing animal fat in general will reduce risk.   Saturated fats should generally be avoided. Good fats include omega 3 fatty acids as found in fish and fish oil, seal oil, nuts like almonds and walnuts, and seeds like sesame and sunflower.   Our ancestors ate equal amounts of omega 3 and omega 6 fats and seldom got cancer. Also very good for you are the omega 9 oils in extra virgin grade cold-pressed olive oil – and this one can stand up to the heat of cooking.

- Protein - organic or chemical free red meat from wild game, or animals raised by traditional herding methods (i.e. grass-fed) is permissible in small portions, for occassional intake. Eating feedlot animals fed on corn silage, growth hormones and stimulants will feed the growth of tumors. Fermented soy products are good, as are true free-range organic eggs and fresh wild fish. Soy protein powder is a good supplement for maintaining vitality and blood sugar balance. Milk whey protein has amino acids which can increase the powerful cancer-killing antioxidant glutathione.

- Sugar - when you eat a lot of simple sugars and refined starches there is a rapid rise in the blood glucose sugar, and a rise in insulin and insulin-like growth factors (IGF). This causes the growth rate of the tumor cells to surge forward for several hours. Choose foods with a low glycemic index and ensure adequate protein.   Eat regularly of wholesome traditional foods, supplement the mineral chromium and antioxidants like vitamins C and E daily.

- Regular physical exercise – is associated with reduced risk of many cancers, and is associated with a sense of well-being and positive quality of life. Exercise fights obesity and moves stagnant blood. Physical activity promotes restful sleep and reduces fatigue. Exercise improves the immune system. All cancer is a failure of the immune system.

- Fiber - A substantial intake of fiber is associated with reduced risk of various cancers. The first priority is lots of fresh vegetables. Whole grain products and fresh organic fruit are probably of some benefit. I prescribe 2 tablespoons daily of fresh-ground flaxseed, and a tablespoon or two of psyllium seed husks. These are easily taken in juice or cereal.

- Xenobiotics - synthetic chemicals, drugs, dyes, food additives, pesticides, herbicides, hormones, animal and plant growth stimulators, tobacco, smog, alcohol and a host of other foreign and non-nutritive compounds we breath, drink and eat are cancer promoters. It is good for us and the planet to reduce our intake of poisons. Choose natural houshold cleaners, personal hygiene products, and other consumables. Keep the liver detoxification systems in top shape with milk thistle, dandelion, beet, and parsley. Take vitamin C and grapeseed extract as antioxidant chemoprotectants.

- Beverages - drink freely of pure water, organic green tea, and red bush (rooibos) tea. For variety try teas of red clover blossoms, graviola leaf, or taheebo bark. Some like *Essiac* or *Flor-Essence*.

- Antioxidants - take selenium, vitamins A, C & E, and grapeseed extract. Whole foods such as beets, fresh greens, tomatoes, the cabbage family, garlic, onions, blueberries, apples, brown rice, etc. provide complexes of antioxidants such as lycopene and lutein, and anticancer compounds such as chlorophyll, flavones, bioflavenoids and polyphenols.

- Calcium and Vitamin D - the modern-era agricultural based diet is actually deficient in calcium. Take with vitamin D3 for best absorption.

- Radiation - avoid sunburn. Minimize exposure to ionizing radiation. Aloe vera is a good mild sunblocker, and like Rosa mosqueta, heals radiation injury.

- Detoxify - see a qualified naturopathic physician for an annual focused personal cleansing program. This may be repeated as needed, but detox is mandatory after chemotherapy.

- Stress management - relaxation and positivity heal. Meditation, prayer, spiritual practices, art, music, and exercise are a great part of a life well spent. Attention should be given to positive and wholesome mental hygiene as well as to nurturing family and positive relationships.

These are the supplements I take daily, for good health and prevention of disease:

Vital Victoria 1-a-day Multivitamin with Minerals Capsule

Vital Victoria Natural Vitamin E - 800 I.U.

Vital Victoria Vitamin C - 1,000 mg

Vital Victoria Grapeseed Extract - 200 mg

Vital Victoria Calcium & Magnesium Citrates with Vitamin D - 2 capsules

AOR standardized gingko biloba extract - 200 mg

AOR Co-Enzyme Q-10 - 100 mg

AOR R-alpha lipoic acid - 100 mg

AOR Fermented Soy Protein Powder - 1 tablespoon

Vitazan   MSM - 1000 mg

Vitazan Plant Source Digestive Enzymes - 1 capsule

Vitazan Plant Sterols & Sterolins - 1 capsule

Vitazan Organic Fresh-ground Flaxseed - 1 tablespoon

Psyllium husks - 1 Tablespoon

Terra Nova Omega 3 Seal Oil - 2 grams

Wu Cha Seng Siberian Ginseng - 4 tablets

Pine Tree Royal Jelly and Ginseng - 2 capsules

I also take a weekly immune tonic: Dolisos Thymuline 9CH - 3 pellets

Vital Victoria products are compounded by a licensed pharmacist.

Chapter Twenty-One - RESEARCH METHODS & SCIENTIFIC EVIDENCE

Evidence-based medicine is the clinical distillation of applications from a database of academic and theoretical research science as well as a range of clinical trials.

Useful data arises from ethical studies that are reproducible, valid and reported factually.

A scientific study should establish if there is a cause and effect between a variable and a given disease or its treatment.

To sort the appropriate data from the deluge of science-like scribblings requires a critical eye. Up to 90% of medical drug studies have serious biases and design flaws, often due to contaminating commercial interests. Editors of scientific and medical journals have recently called for full disclosure of any involvement by the authors with commercial interests, and freedom for scientists to publish all their negative findings.

QUASI-EXPERIMENTAL DESIGNS
- simple surveys, anecdotal, indirect associations
- descriptive, raises questions
- correlational study, without a comparison group
- experimental, without control for confounding variables
- do not rule out alternative hypotheses
- artifactual, spurious, or biased associations
- self-selected or constitutionally disposed subjects
- *in vitro*
- *in vivo* animal studies

NULL HYPOTHESIS
Null studies are designed to prove the hypothesis is wrong, by testing all conceivable alternative variables. Failure to find another valid explanation can be good evidence for the default interpretation.

It is a marker of pseudoscience to have a "hypothesis which cannot be false"- in other words, which cannot be stated in a way which is open to testing that it is erroneous. Religious ideologies are classic examples of theories which are irrefutable, and therefore unscientific.

Irrational and chaotic subjects such as emotions, psychology, faith, dreams, mind and experience are beyond the scientific method. Testable models just are not as complex as real life. Sorry science buffs, its not as simple as you may like.

GOOD EXPERIMENTAL DESIGNS

- randomization of all variables
- confounding variables controlled by matching, blocking, or specific stratification of subjects
- blinded assignment and assessment
- ethics approved by independent review - confidentiality, safety and informed consent.
- analytical, addresses the hypothesis and objectives stated
- data from all cases are reported
- methods are detailed
- rigorous, "necessary and sufficient" logic
- diagnosis follows accepted standards and methods
- outcome measurement follows accepted standards and methods
- new therapies are compared to placebo, no treatment and to recognized treatments
- disclosure of toxicity data and adverse events
- statistically significant results - has the power of large numbers
- peer review of the evidence

The "gold standard" in medical research since 1945 is the placebo-controlled double-blind randomized clinical trial. A series of significant and irrefutable Phase 3 trials of this type are required to prove a therapy to a high scientific standard.

Many alternative therapies have come up against a bureaucratic wall demanding proof of safety and effectiveness to this expensive, organizationally complex and ethically questionable standard. It is scientifically reasonable in preliminary studies to substitute "historical controls" for patients receiving placebo. In fact before anyone will pay the big dollars for big studies, many smaller scale and less rigorous trial designs will have to be used to probe for truth. Consider that most new agents are only given to patients who are not responsive to the mainstream therapies. Only the terminal, advanced, end-stage and very damaged cases are given access. This is rarely a fair test, particularly of natural agents which are gentle, normalizing, and rely on activating the self-healing mechanisms of the body. To only throw the actively dying patients into the studies of alternative and complementary medicines will assure we only see poor outcomes most of the time. Such is the nature of very advanced cancer, it is very harsh and mostly fatal. When you are dealing with a stage of disease that is almost invariably fatal, why add the cruelty of a placebo, knowingly withholding any known active therapy from these poor people? The Chinese have always considered such practices to be unethical and unbecoming of a physician, and they have convinced me it is not always the best way to make progress in medicine.

The policies of the National Research Council regarding the investigation of a novel cancer therapy:

- full disclosure of the chemical formula of the medication, or if a full chemical analysis is not available, the exact method of preparation.
- complete laboratory and clinical records.
- microscopic confirmation of the diagnosis of cancer in test subjects
- accepted medical evidence of the arrest or disappearance of cancer attributed to the medication.
- detailed description of any other treatment prior to the investigational treatment.
- all data on doseage and posology (how a medicine is given)
- all data on laboratory findings prior, during and subsequent to the investigational treatment.
- the National Cancer Institute reserves the right to publish its findings, and to decide when and if any further investigation is justified based on the evidence presented.

These seem reasonable on the surface, but why have so many sincere physicians who have advanced ideas based on careful clinical observation of results with new therapies encountered a consistent pattern of abuse, denial, bigoted rejection of their ideas without testing, or decried the few tests performed as being biased and unfair? There is something deeper here than a conspiracy to prevent a cure for cancer. My observations of the medical, drug and science industry is that it has accepted a basic world view generations ago which blind it to natural medicines. It is intensely frustrating to see medicines which clearly create health rejected from clinical practice simply because they do not instantly cure disease.

The underlying concept of one specific medicine for each disease began with the Eclectic school of herbalists in America, from whom naturopathic doctors have inherited a great deal of their botanical medicine. As scientists looked for the 'active principle' in complex plant drugs, they indeed found these concentrated chemicals had specific targets in the body, altering enzymes, changing genetic expression, and so on. They then began to screen millions of chemicals for such dramatic and fast effects on cells in test tubes and on animals such as mice. For example, the Madagascar periwinkle flower was processed, hundreds of chemicals extracted, separated and purified. Several were found to inhibit cancer cells, and two of these have become standard chemotherapy drugs Vincristine and Vinblastine. It is important to note that only these two substances became drugs. Several other compounds in this plant fight cancer, but have never been developed into therapies. How many other compounds in this plant might have more subtle effects, not seen in all cell lines - and only a few types of cancer cells are used for screening - or not seen in mice, or not seen immediately, but whose value would be expressed slowly as the immune system is strengthened, the liver and organs are cleansed, or some other health building process occurs?

There is no system in place to test for medicines which are non-specific stimulants of the healing process, tonifers, balancers and harmonizers. These are exactly the kind of medicines Traditional Chinese Medicine and Naturopathic Medicine use.

SENSIBLE STATISTICAL INTERPRETATION

A positive outcome in a study forms a positive statistical association that such a result can be obtained in your practice with actual patients. Probabilities with statistical significance do not always mean biological and clinical significance. There is the possible role of chance in complex systems.

- *Chi square test* measures the correlation of a trait or its absence with a disease .
- *t-test* compares the mean level of a quantitative attribute in disease and control groups.
- analysis of covariance
- regression analysis
- multivariate analysis

THE ELUSIVE "NORMAL" CASE

- individuals vary widely and in complex ways
- normal ranges are often based on standard deviations from the mean, a mathematical precept with no biological meaning.
- homeostasis tends to produce normative values
- anything can happen when a system destabilizes

No patient is a textbook case, just like the one before. There are probabilities we can quote from medical studies, but we all know exceptional cases. There are cures, even in late stages of mortal diseases. Chaos theory predicts in complex systems there will be sudden quantum shifts to new states, with small inputs sometimes producing massive changes in outcomes.

Bernie Siegel, MD is a cancer surgeon and author who certainly had a bright idea when he decided to spend more of his time looking at what the survivors of cancer did that was different from the ones who perished. They had love, hope and faith in miracles.

PHASE 1 STUDY

- small group of patients
- focus is on the pharmacokinetics and toxicity, not how useful it is
- identifies the types of adverse reactions
- determines the maximum tolerated dose
- dose is slowly ramped up until toxicity occurs

PHASE 2 STUDY

- larger scale, more participants and longer trial
- control groups are added
- standardized dose and posology (method of delivery)
- tests for efficacy of an intervention

PHASE 3 STUDY

- blinded
- larger, longer, often multi-centric (at several institutions)
- compares one intervention to others, such as the new therapy against an established treatment as well as against a control group

META-ANALYSIS

Analysis and correlation of data from multiple independent studies.
A virtual study based on several existing data pools.

DESIRABLE CHARACTERISTICS OF A SCIENTIFIC CLINICAL TRIAL

A multi-agency federal USA group developed these qualifying criteria:

- the principal purpose of the trial is to test whether the intervention potentially improves the participants' health outcomes.
- the trial is well-supported by available scientific and medical information or it is intended to clarify or establish the health outcomes of interventions already in common clinical use.
- the trial does not unjustifiably duplicate existing studies.
- the trial design is appropriate to answer the research question being asked
- the trial is sponsored by a credible institution or organization or conducted by an individual capable of executing the trial successfully.
- the trial is in compliance with regulations related to the protection of human subjects.
- the trial is conducted according to appropriate standards of scientific integrity.

OTHER CRITERIA OF GOOD RESEARCH

- disclosure of collaborators, consultants, contractual arrangements.
- identifies and properly acknowledges work already published - a literature review.
- approval by an Institutional Review Board (IRB).
- conclusive evidence can only be obtained from well-characterized agents tested in suitable cohorts and using scientific rigor to evaluate efficacy based on reliable intermediate biomarkers of cancer.

EMPIRICAL SCIENCE

My training in modern physics taught me about relativity of such things as space, time, probability and uncertainty, the role of the observer in the outcome of events, the multi-dimensionality of reality, and the chaos that often underlies order. Life is even more complex than medicine.

I believe in the principle of *Vis Medicatrix Naturae* the healing power of Nature.

I understand we are created in the divine spirit which is manifesting by expressing and experiencing itself in ways that are non-linear, non-local and yet coherent.

Medicine has made many blunders expecting all patients to get more benefit than harm from any single 'standardized' treatment. Cause and effect relationships are synchronous only when they occupy the same piece of what Einstein called *space-time*. This is relative, subjective, the very interaction depending on thought, feeling and awareness.

Localization is responsible for the perception of time progressing as an arrow. I travel every week on a bus. The landscape "unfolds" before me, along a predictable time-line. The landscape is for all intents and purposes everywhere, but as I am not, I experience a particular series of chaotic current events against a familiar background which changes only much more gradually. My "reality" depends on where my focus is.

Chaos theory predicts complex systems - which is any with three or more variables acting upon it - such as the human organism - are subject to a wide range of possibilities, with very small inputs generating very large changes when repeated often. I have seen this with many wholistic therapies such as homeopathy, acupuncture, Reiki and in all the psychological methods.

I believe the real power is in feelings like Love and in Truth and in Consciousness. Restoring meaningful symbols to a human is a creative act which can save a life. All it takes sometimes is a change in perspective. Belief and perception create experience.

Is there really any "objective" truth out there for our scientists to measure? The search for infallible data is subject to so many unreal conditions that it is always prone to the fallibility of statistical error and dispute. In fact all events have a context. Artificially removing context alters the meaning of the event and our experience of it.

I work from as much of a rational and scientific basis as I can when it comes to anatomy, biochemistry, pathology, and other medical databases. My thoughts are informed by data. However, I have emotions, feelings, and beliefs which interpret the expression of what I experience.

Some of my medical beliefs come from an empirical system which looks at the constitution and higher organization of the body. Some come from humanistic psychology. I do believe in energy healing. It seems there are medical truths expressed by whole people, whole foods, whole plants, and whole networks of living things which are just not getting studied, given the current interpretation of what is "scientific".

The era of focussing on chemotherapy drugs has had its run, the results have been very limited, have now reached a plateau, and it is time to try a new model.

I believe the plants and foods discussed in this book, if tested by appropriate methods on human beings, will provide great progress in cancer care. We cannot let these treasures be turned into commodities and nihilistic medicines which do great harm.
I do not support testing isolates, synthetic versions, and single agents. I do not support mouse abuse, or withholding safe treatments from cancer patients.

It is essential to nourish, nurture, cleanse and heal every patient to the limit of our skill and knowledge. We do need drug medicine to deal with emergencies, but we also need natural remedies to live in harmony with our biology. How did it come to be that safe and gentle therapies are only considered after the cancer patient is subject to very harsh medicines and the advancing disease has wreaked havoc? How is it that we consider it normal to ignore general tonics, nutrtives and cleansers while undergoing stressful and risky treatments for cancer? The scientists feel a need to keep it simple, but the bigger priority for the patient is keeping alive - and whose life is it anyway?

Life on this planet has found amazing ways to survive. By studying whole foods, whole plants, wholistic methods, and individual patients, we can tap into a variety of new treatment concepts. Working with life-enhancing methods, not just cancer-killing therapies, we will survive the cancer epidemic.

The drug medicine industrial complex, from the office of the general practitioner to the big institutes and research hospitals, are an exclusive club dedicated to their own self-perpetuation. Individual doctors may have ethics and humanitarian principles - however their masters generally seem intent on power and money.

Novel ideas are not just resisted in the interest of being rigorous and prudent, they are often attacked with a level of ferocity that is shameful. Where it serves them, such as when an independent doctor helps a patient, all of a sudden cancer becomes hard to define, treatment outcomes become impractical to measure, and theories become incomprehensible. Cured cases are declared to have been mis-diagnosed. However, based on the same diagnostic techniques it is ethical to give treatments which can be fatal. So can they only diagnose properly when the patient will get orthodox treatment?

Are we to suffer on, losing ground against cancer, until someone finds a way to commercialize every plant on the planet and all the DNA of everything else too? It is sad how often an innovation from a fertile open mind has been denied for years, then one day it is moved from Quack to Proven when it is put to the profit of the current dominant players in the medical industry.

Great thinkers in this field, and there have been many, have too often been treated with malfesiance and duplicity, and if their ideas cannot be converted or stolen for profit, they are destroyed. The public willingly pours almost limitless money into research, and it is entirely spent on drugs owned by for-profit corporations or methods which are compatible with current medical hardware and expertise. The fact that the war on cancer has been a losing game does not deter them from maintaining the status quo at all costs. It is estimated that a new drug costs over $125 million US dollars to research to the point where it can be approved as a new therapy. That process takes about 10 years.
Drug companies are not about to let into the game cheaper and safer natural products which have cost a lot less in research investment. They will not tolerate reduced return on their patented drugs and procedures.

The medical mafia is alive and well in Canada, and abroad. They are not evil, they are just self-serving. I think every person can be corrupted by power and money, and will revert to a tribalistic isolation to keep hold of what they have. I may be a minority in my opinion that natural medicines are good. I do not have to consume drug medicine, nor do I have to accept that drug medicine can consume all the research and health care dollars.

The conduct of the mainstream institutions attempting to do alternative cancer research has mostly been either ineffective or disinterested in real outcomes the public is waiting for. Krebiozen, anti-neoplastons and so many other remedies brought forward in good faith by reputable clinicians and scientists have never been tested fairly, nor repeatedly, and then ruled upon in a timely way, as good science demands. They say "we just don't know", then expect people to follow their advice about the issue. Is "evidence based medical practice" guided by hunches, suspicions and fears? If it is decided before testing "It can't work", then that is "psychic science" and I refuse to allow it to pass as real science. No real hypothesis is untestable.

It is very disturbing to see real opportunities for controlling this horrendous disease being subject to a cynical black-out, and access denied. How many lives have been squandered over greed, jealousy and outright stupidity by the accepted scientific community? Far too many in that group are sheep who have given up the power of objective and dispassionate reasoning for the lure of lucre, most of which of course flows through the mainstream of humanity. What most people settle for is what is ruled safe and generally agreed upon. That is a very subjective call. There is a lot of good knowledge and medicine that ends up left outside that box.

Scientific fundamentalism is as dangerous as the worst religious fanaticism. That attitude dooms millions of cancer sufferers today, and into the foreseeable future, to more of the "same old same old".

I urge adults to demand their sovereign right to free choice, to access treatments offered in good faith, which have low risk of harm, and a history of therapeutic value. I understand we have soveriegnty in what we believe as an inherent right due to us from our creation in spirit or divinity. We do not expect the science industry to be able or willing to bless all our options as proven to a high degree of certainty. Life is just like that, a little risky, and the consequences are ours to bear. I do not give up the right to choose my health care to anyone else, not even my doctor. I have the right to be wrong, and face the consequences.

"Today's mighty oak is just yesterday's nut that held its ground".

Reasonable people want to access the state of the art, not just the state of the science, of medicine. I have a deep conviction that cancer can be overcome in many ways, at many levels. Just like the rest of life, it is a personal journey.

Don't ever give up, because naturally there's hope!

BIBLIOGRAPHY & READING LIST

- *Clinical Oncology*, American Cancer Society, 2000
- *Robbins Pathologic Basis of Disease*, Sixth edition, R. Cotran, V. Kumar, & T. Collins, W.B. Saunders Company
- *Cancer & Natural Medicine - a Textbook of Basic Science and Clinical Research*, John Boik, 1996, Oregon Medical Press
- *Natural Compounds in Cancer Therapy*, John Boik, 2001, Oregon Medical Press
- *You Don't Have to Die*, Harry Hoxsey, N.D., 1956 Milestone Books
- *The Cancer Industry -Unravelling the Politics*, Ralph W. Moss, 1989, Paragon
- *A Family Guide - Coping with Chemotherapy Using Homeopathy*, Laura Fenton, 2003, Health Harmony Books.
- *An Introduction to Integrated Healing - Participants' guide to self-care, healthful nutrition, vitamins, supplements, complementary medical therapies and healing*, Center for Integrated Care, 1998
- *Third Opinion: An International Directory to Alternative Therapy Centres for the Treatment and Prevention of Cancer and Other Degenerative Diseases*, Second edition, J. M. Fink, 1992; Avery Publishing Group.
- *A Guide to Unconventional Cancer Therapies*, Ontario Breast Cancer Information Exchange Project, 1994
- *Breast Cancer - What you should know (but may not be told) about prevention, diagnosis and treatment*, Steve Austin, N.D. and Cathy Hitchcock, M.S.W., 1994, Prima Health Publishing
- *Breast Cancer - The Complete Guide*, Third edition, Yashar Hirshaut & Peter Pressman, 2000, Bantam Books.
- *Breast Cancer - A Nutritional Approach*, Carlton Fredericks, Ph.D., 1977, Grosset & Dunlap
- *Beating Cancer with Nutrition*, Patrick Quillan, 1994, Nutrition times Press.
- *Paleolithic Prescription*, Easton, Shostak & Konner, 1988; Harper & Row
- *Secrets to Great Health*, Jonn Matsen, N.D., 2001, Prima Publishing
- *The Schwarzbein Principle*, Diana Schwarzbein, MD, 1999, Health Communications.
- *A Holistic Approach to Cancer Therapy*, Wolfgang Woeppel, 1995, Pascoe
- *Love, Medicine & Miracles* - Lessons learned about self-healing from a surgeon's experience with exceptional patients, Bernie. S. Siegel, M.D., 1986, Harper & Row
- *Homeopathic Medical Repetory*, Robin Murphy, N.D., 1993; Hahnemann Academy of North America.

- *The Cancer Epidemic: Shadow of the Conquest of Nature*, Gotthard Booth, 1974, Edwin Mellen Press
- *Cancer Therapy - the Independent Consumer's Guide to Non-toxic Treatment and Prevention*, Ralph Moss, Equinox Press
- *Healthy Fats For Life - Preventing and treating common health problems with essential fatty acids*, L. Vanderhaege, K. Karst, 2003, Quarry Health Books
- *How to Prevent and Treat Cancer with Natural Medicine*, Michael Murray, Tim Birdsall, Joseph E. Pizzorno & Paul Reilly, 2002, Riverhead Books
- *Cancer and Vitamin C*, Ewan Cameron & Linus Pauling, 1979, Linus Pauling Institute of Science and Medicine
- *Cancer as a Turning Point*, Lawrence LeShan, Penguin Press
- *Nutritional Management of Cancer Patients*, Abby S. Block, Aspen Publishers
- *Everyone's Guide to Cancer Therapy*, M. Dollinger, E. Rosebaum, & G. Cable, Andrews-McMeel Publishers
- *The Wheatgrass Book*, Ann Wigmore, 'Doctor of Natural Laws', 1985, Avery Publishing Group.
- *Cancer Principles and Practices*, V. DeVita, S. Hellman,& S. Rosenberg, Lipincott-Raven Publishers
- *Handbook of Cancer Chemotherapy*, Roland T. Skeel, Lipincott.
- *Manual of Clinical Oncology*, D. Casciato & B. Lowitz, Little Brown
- *Primer of Epidemiology*, Gary Friedman, 1980, McGraw-Hill
- *Foundations of Epidemiology*, A. Lilienfeld,1976, Oxford U. Press
- *FDA Supplement Warnings - Misleading, Exaggerated or Unproven*, Zoltan Rona, June/July 1998, Health Naturally
- *Increasing and Improving Research in Complementary and Alternative Medicine*, Carlo Calabrese, 2000, NIH Office of Alternative Medicine.
- *The Cancer Blackout - A history of denied and suppressed remedies*, Maurice Natenberg, 1959, Regent House.
- *The Medical Mafia - How to get out of it alive and take back our health & wealth*, Ghislaine Lanctot, 2002 edition, self-published.
- *Cancer - A Healing Crisis - the whole-body approach to cancer therapy*, Jack Tropp, 1980, Exposition Press.
- *The Healing of Cancer - The cures, the cover-ups and the solution now*, Barry Lynes, 1989, Marcus Books.
- *The Tao of Medicine*, Stephen Fulder, 1982, Destiny Books.
- *Cancer Treatment with Fu Zheng Pei Ben Principle*, Pan Mingji, et al, 1992, Fujian Science & Technology Publishing House.

RECOMMENDED JOURNALS

- Cancer
- Nutrition & Cancer
- Journal of Clinical Oncology
- Journal of the National Cancer Institute
- Cancer Research
- Integrative Cancer Care
- American Journal of Clinical Nutrition
- Alternative Medicine Review
- International Journal of Cancer
- Clinical Pearls
- Anticancer Research
- Townsend Letter for Doctors & Their Patients

WEB RESOURCES

- www.cancerfacts.com
- www.nci.nih.gov
- www.cancernet.nci.nih.gov/clinpdq
- www.cancer.org   American Cancer Society 1-800-ACS-2345
- www.cdc.gov.org/cancer
- www.bccancer.bc.ca
- www.y-me.org
- www.asco.org
- www.Medscape.com - oncology database
- www.graviola.org

CLINIC COORDINATES
Vital Victoria Naturopathic Clinic
3534 Quadra Street
Victoria, BC
Canada   V8X 1H2
Phone: (250) 386 – 3534   Fax: (250) 386 - 3500

INDEX

Carotenoids 42,51,52,58,76,81,146,151,177,187,192,193,203

Cartilage 83

Caspase enzymes 18,73,74,108,114

Castor oil pack 55

Catechin 28,38,93,145

Cat's claw 38,62,100,135,146,188,200

Cellular adhesion 13,17,25,32,83,85,100,108

Cervical cancer 15,31,104,122,127,186

Chamomile 45,50,52

Chemotherapy 46 to 54,107

Chlorophyll 8,45,58,72,100,132,203

Chromium 60,202

Cisplatin 51

Cod liver oil 45,50,61,69,86,146,147,176,189,200

Coenzyme Q-10 50,51,52,81,100,146,195

Coffee 24,76,85,102,135

Coley's toxins 59,124,129

Colorectal cancer 17,30,34,35,61,66,67,68,76,77,79,93,95,96,98109,127,137,138,
            150,173-177

Comedo variant 156

Conjugated linoleic acid CLA 26,45,49,67,145,146 ,185

Constipation 45,49,97,117,118,135,138

Constitutional hydrotherapy 55

Contact inhibition 13,25,67

Copper 28,75

Corynebacterium parvum vaccine 129,148

COX – see cyclooxygenases

C-reactive protein 30,61,63

Cribriform variant 156

Cryosurgery 168,190,192

Curcumin 24,32,38,42,47,52,58,79,92,93,96,106,135,145,146,
            147,171,177,184,189,190,193,195,200,201

Cyclins 16,156

Cyclooxygenases COX 31,32,42,63,78,98,104,114,115,135,145,173,182,193

Cyclophosphamide 51,107,112

Cytochrome p-450 32,73

Cytokines 14,17,30,30,53,62,63,81,85,97,99,100,107,129,138,200

Cytology 33

Cytotoxins 5,39,67,74,76,78,67,90,95,97,98,99,101,104,107,108 ,127,130,146,201

Dang gui lu hui 112,200

Death ligands 73

Dehydration 44

Desquamation 43

Detoxification 21,48,55,68,75,99,102,109,117,134,135,195,203

Fiber 8,45,49,58,66,148,151,162,173,177,203
Fibrin 28,85,100,114
Fibrosis 40,42
Fish otolith formula 113,196
5-alpha reductase 69,93,108
Flaxseed 55,146,147,148,162,171,188,203
5-Fluorouracil 52,107,159
Folate/folic acid 16,45,50,51,52
#42's 49,97
Free radicals – see Reactive Oxygen Species
Fu zheng sheng jin
Gamma linolenic acid oils GLA 53,67,146,162,172,195
Ganoderma – see Reishi mushroom
Garlic 32,37,54,56,58,83,170,172
Gastric – see Stomach cancer
Gastro-intestinal cancer 34,40
Gemcitabine 53,191
Genestein 24,28,42,52,79,84,96,97,145,146,191
Genetics 11,13
Gerson diet 57,59,65,66
Ginger root 44,45,49
Gingko biloba 37,44,49,51,138,185
Ginseng 37,43,44,45,48,50,54,63,98,106,108,109,110,111,146,185,190,200,201
Gleason score 166
Glutathione 24,42,44,45,47,49,51,52,55,64,75,82,95,107,146,147,148,177,184,
        190,202
Goose blood tablets 112,200
Goserlin 159
Gotu kola 38,103
Grading 23,154,166175,182
Grapefruit 54
Grapeseed extract 32,55,75,92,95,135,146,147,177,181,190,193,195,203
Graviola 98,105,146,147,190,191,203
Green tea 28,32,42,44,52,61,62,79,92,93,94,95,96,138,145,146,147,
        151,162,163,164,172,184,190,191,193
Growth inhibitors 15,17,20,77,82,101,102
Growth factors (promoters) 15,16,17,19,25,27,31,60,65,75,97,155
Haelen 64,84
Hand-foot syndrome 50,52
HCG human chorionic gonadotrophin 34
Heat shock proteins 19,77,79,82,96,124,146,177
Helicobacter pylori 189,197
Hemorrhage 36,44,113,137,138
Heparin 26,27,145

Hepatocellular carcinoma – see Liver cancer
Herbicides 31,58,75,149
Herbotox 55,134,147
HER-2/neu gene 31,150,158,161
Herceptin 161
HETE – see Lipoxygenases
Histamine 28,97,130,148
Hodgkin's disease 15,21,40,102
Homeopathy 3,44,45,49,118,128,135,136,138,141,178,181,193,195
Homocysteine 16
Homotoxicology 21,118
Hormone modulators 146
Horse chestnut 104,106,138
Hoxsey tonic 45,49,53,65,76,87,88,89,90,147,190,191,193,195
Human papilloma virus 15,104,186
Hydrazine sulphate 63
Hydrochloric acid 43,48
Hydrogenated fats 32
Hydrogen peroxide 74,78,122,130
Hypercalcemia 53,69,139,140
Hypericum 37,43,53,54
Hyperthermia 19,124
Hypoxia 14,27,28,31,34,40,42
Immune evasion 29
Immune therapies 19,21,27,30,54,59,64,67,77,79,81,83,97,98,99,100,103,104,105,
            106,107,111,112,115,116,117,121,123,124,127,128,135,146
Immunosuppression 15,22,30,31,32,36,38,47,104,130
Indirubin 201
Indole-3-carbinol 58,82,146,151,162,164,187
Induction 20
Infection 36,43,48,100,102,104,128,131,136
Inflammation 14,24,28,30,31,32,38,43,91,96,97,98,99,100,102,
          104,106,109,110,114,115,117,122,131,134,135,142,146
in situ 19,22,165
Insulin 28,31,57,60,61,62,65,67,76,108,112,133,165,170,173,177
Insulin-like growth factors 16,19,61,69,76,93,158,165,172,173
            177,190,202
Interferons 38,78,99,104,129,130
Interleukins 19,28,30,31,32,61,62,63,67,74,79,81,96,102,104,107
            108,110,116,124,129,130
Internal dissolution pills 109,147,181,190,191,195
Invasion 20,23,31,32,36,84,104,108
Iodine 58,59,65,66,77,89,146,147
IP6 – see Phytic acid
Iron 24,43,65,137

Lymphoma 15,21,22,30,35,47,100,102,104,112,114, 127,136,137,138,140
Magnesium 32,65,81,85
Magnetics 126
Maitake PSK 42,146,148
Mammograms 152
Mammastatin 154
Marijuana 44,49
Marrow Plus 43,48
Mastectomy 156,157
Mastic gum 189
Medical mafia 212
Melanoma 17,30,77,93,103,127,129,130,193
Melatonin 42,44,45,49,51,52,53,62,80,108,126,138,146,147,162,171,177,181,184,
        188,195,200
Menopausal status 155
Metallo-proteinase enzymes 31,93
Metallothionen 65
Metastasis 20,22,23,26,28,31,32,36,37,38,78,85,92,100,101,104,
        108,114,139,145
Methotrexate 52,107
Methylation of DNA 16
Methylmalonic acid 16
Methylsulphonylmethane MSM 122,193
Mibi scan 152
Microcluster water 55,126
Milk thistle 42,44,50,51,62,134,146,147,163,172,184,190
Miraluma scan 152
Mistletoe 24,87,99,145,146,190,191
Mitosis 16,40
Mitomycin 112
Modified citrus pectin 26,36,37,38,145,172
Momordica 45
Monoclonal antibodies 27,30,35
Morbidity 10
Mortality 10
Mouth sores/mucositis 45,50,118
MRI scan 153,166
MRV 129,148
MUC1 mucin 191
Multidrug resistance 78,108
Mung bean sprouts 54
Mushroom polysaccharides 107,132,146,148,184
Mutations 13,19,20,47,68,84,92
Myeloma 35,130,200

Ping xiao pian 110,147
Pishen Fang 111,190
p21 gene 66,78,108,177
p27 gene 150,165
p53 gene 17,47,66,75,76,77,81,82,95,108,146,150,1 69,182
p63 gene 189
Phenethylisothiocyanates 58
Phytic acid 66
Phytolacca 43,48,90
Platelet-derived growth factor 16,19,155,161,199
Pneumonitis 44,47
Po Chai 45,49
Podophyllum 51,87,89,103
Polyerga spleen peptides 51,54,130,146,148
Polygonum 95,114,201
Poly-MVA lipoic palladium 82
Polyphenols 8,58,77,92,93,146,172,203
Polyunsaturated fatty acids 68,73
Potassium 8,58,59,65,85,88,136
Potassium iodide – see Iodine
Prayer 38
Proanthocyanidins – see Grapeseed extract
Probiotics 38,45,49,68,142,1 48,151,173,177
Progesterone 31,32,58,63,70,150,157,163,169,170,186,188
Progesterone receptor status 155
Progression 20,32,96
Prolactin 81,163,165
Proliferation 20,23,31,65,72,79,81,83,109,111,114,125,166
Prostaglandins 14,28,30,31,32,63,64,67,78,79, 91,97,100,139
Prostate cancer 34,61,65,68,76,88,93,98,102,114,127,137,
        150,164-172
PSA Prostate specific antigen 34,165,166
Prostatectomy 168
Proteolytic enzymes 15,25,38,75,85,86,131,136,146,147,148
Pseudoginseng – see Yunnan Baiyao
Psychotherapy 117,119,120,132,177
Psyllium husks 55,66,68,146,148,203
Pulmonary tonic tablets 114
Quercitin 24,32,42,47,50,51,52,53,77,79,85,96,100,145,147,160,163,177,184,
        188,193,201
Radiation 39,122
Radiation protectants 42,76,98,100,107
Radiofrequency ablation 125,190
Radiosensitizers 3,42,98,109,113,124
Radon gas 178
ras gene protein 16,31,61,161,177,198

Rattlesnake plantain 105
Reactive oxygen species ROS 14,20,39,40,62,72,73,93,104,113,130
Red clover blossoms 53,97,103,138,203
Redox (reduction/oxidation) 14,72,75,77
Reiki 1,117
Reishi mushroom 38,45,54,63,107,109,112,146,148,188
Renal –see Kidney cancer
Research methods 205
Response to therapy standards 144
Reticuloendothelial immune cells 79,96,103,105,108,113,128,13 1
Retroviruses 14,15
Revici 70,71
Rife ray 123
Roiboos tea 95,203
Rosa mosqueta 43,203
Rosemary 54,56,135,146,163
Royal jelly 44,45,50,54,63,108,115
Rubia 115
S-adenosylmethionine 16
S-phase analysis 155
Salt 38,44,45,49,50,89,109,113
Salvia 114
Saposhnikovia 105
Sarcoma 79,96,127
Saw palmetto 170
Scarring – see Fibrosis
Scintography 152
Scutellaria 32,109,135
SeaBand 44,49
Seagest protein 64
Selenium 14,42,51,52,55,65,75,81,85,123,146,147,148,164,172,173,184,
        188,190,191,203
Sesame oil 43,48
714X 123
Sex hormone binding globulins 84,114,158,162
SF734 189
Shark liver oil 28,42,43,48,68,145
Shen mai zhu she ye 110
Shen xue tang 111,190
Shih Chuan Da Bu Wan 43,48,54,110,137,146,190,200
Shiitake mushroom 48,146,148
Shikonin 28,145
Sho-saiko-to 111
Siberian ginseng – see Eleutherococcus
Si jun zi tang 111,190
Skin cancer 8,22,67,69,90,94,102,103,192,193

ACKNOWLEDGEMENTS & THANKS

Thank you Egon Milinkovitch for healing me, which allowed me to walk this path.

My brothers John and Jim and sister Norma helped pull me through a rough start, and continue to amaze me.

I am ever grateful to my dear mother Stella for creating my interest in reading and study, as well as my interest in spirit.

I thank Terry Fox for demonstrating the courage to try to get things moving forward for today's cancer patients.

I thank Dr. John Bastyr, N.D. for his example of the pursuit of knowledge and brevity in communicating it.

I must thank Dr. David Scotten, ND for having me teach Oncology at the Boucher Institute of Naturopathic Medicine, which started me writing.

I am much indebted to my colleagues at Cancer Treatment Centers of America for sharing their advanced knowledge of integrated cancer care.

I give thanks for my daughters Angela, Talia and Tracy, who give me the desire to work hard to make this a better world.

I thank "Nana" Joy DeProy for Lynda and all her family for so much joy in my life.

With all my heart I thank my patients for sharing their lives so freely with me.

Yours in health,

Dr. Neil McKinney, BSc, RAc, ND